MAYO CLINIC

· ·

FIRST-AID GUIDE FOR OUTDOOR ADVENTURES

Neha P. Raukar, M.D., M.S.

MAYO CLINIC | Mayo Clinic Press

Published by Mayo Clinic Press

© 2024 Mayo Foundation for Medical Education and Research (MFMER)

For bulk sales to employers, member groups and health-related companies, contact Mayo Clinic, 200 First St. SW, Rochester, MN 55905, or email SpecialSalesMayoBooks@mayo.edu.

To stay informed about Mayo Clinic Press, please subscribe to our free e-newsletter at MCPress.MayoClinic.org or follow us on social media.

When you purchase Mayo Clinic newsletters and books, proceeds are used to further medical education and research at Mayo Clinic. You not only get answers to your questions on health, you become part of the solution.

ISBN 979-8-887700-36-6

Library of Congress Control Number: 2023942935

Printed in China

MAYO CLINIC PRESS

Medical Editor
Neha P. Raukar, M.D., M.S.

Publisher
Daniel J. Harke

Editor in Chief
Nina E. Wiener

Senior Editor
Karen R. Wallevand

Principal Product Manager
James R. Cahoy

Art Director
Stewart J. Koski

Design Manager
Amanda J. Knapp

Illustration
Steve D. Orwoll
Marty Harris

Contributors
Luke E. Wood, D.O.
Richard C. Winters, M.D.
Matthew Sholl, M.D.

Additional contributions from
Girl Friday Productions, Devon
Frederickson and Rath Indexing

Cover design by
Girl Friday Productions

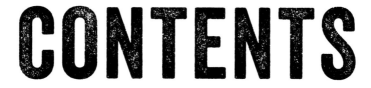

CONTENTS

DEAR FELLOW ADVENTURER,

As a practicing physician in both sports and emergency medicine, I've had the privilege of witnessing the wonders of the great outdoors and the exhilaration that comes with exploring its boundless beauty. The wilderness has a way of captivating our hearts and souls like nothing else can.

However, amidst the thrill and splendor of outdoor escapades, lies an inherent truth — nature, for all its magnificence, can be unforgiving, presenting us with unforeseen challenges and medical emergencies that demand swift and informed action. Whether you're a seasoned adventurer or a beginner stepping into the unknown, being prepared for the unexpected is an absolute must.

That is precisely why we developed this book — your ultimate companion for first aid in the outdoors. It equips you with the essential knowledge and skills to respond effectively to emergencies and handle injuries when medical help isn't readily available.

Preparation is the key in creating enjoyable outdoor pursuits. Whether you're planning a short hike, a camping trip, or embarking on an extended sailing expedition, having the right tools in your mental and physical toolbox can make all the difference in ensuring your safety and the safety of those around you.

In this book, you'll find practical, step-by-step instructions for managing a wide range of injuries and medical emergencies.

From treating common cuts and bruises to handling more serious incidents like fractures and dislocations, each chapter is thoughtfully designed to empower you with the confidence to respond effectively when minutes count.

Within these pages we've also infused the latest insights and best practices drawn from personal experiences in practicing emergency medicine and sports medicine. We hope this knowledge will not only serve as a lifeline in challenging times but also empower you to embrace your adventures with greater awareness and preparedness.

As you embark on your next outdoor expedition, let *Mayo Clinic First-Aid Guide for Outdoor Adventures* be your steadfast companion, providing you with the tools to navigate the unexpected and make the most of your outdoor pursuits. Together, let's make every journey a safe and memorable one.

Wishing you safe travels and unforgettable experiences.

Yours in adventure,

Dr. Neha Raukar

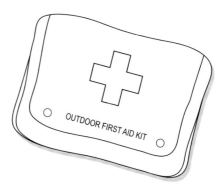

INTRODUCTION

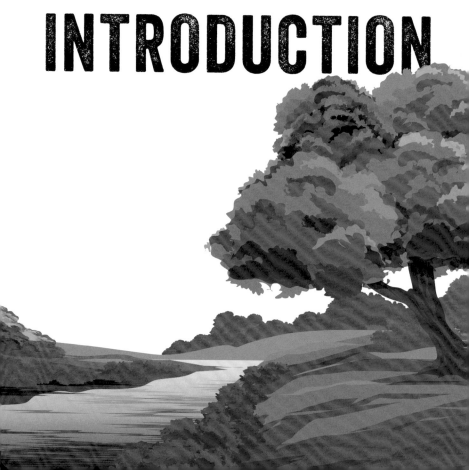

o matter how carefully you plan, things can go wrong in the wilderness. One misstep on an uneven trail and you've sprained your ankle. One water filter left in the car and you risk waterborne illness. Between mosquitoes and blisters, sunburn and splinters, and toxic plants that lurk in the undergrowth, the odds of staying comfortable and safe in the outdoors may begin to feel like trekking through dense, uncharted terrain without a guide.

The good news is, as long as you check the forecast, pack appropriate clothing and gear (including a first-aid kit), research your destination and minimize exploring solo, you'll have an adventure to remember. Still, accidents happen, and when they do, you might be far away from civilization and cell service. No calling 911. You'll have to problem-solve your way out of danger yourself.

Enter: *Mayo Clinic First-Aid Guide for Outdoor Adventures*.

This book covers everything for the open-air enthusiast, from what to pack to how to respond to varying degrees of crisis, including signs and symptoms to look out for and step-by-step treatment instructions. You'll also find prevention tips to help you avoid getting into sticky situations in the first place. The goal? Equipping you with all the tools you might need to address a medical accident in the wilderness. That way, even if things go wrong, you'll know the right steps to respond to any scenario with cool, collected confidence.

WILDERNESS FIRST-RESPONSE STEPS

While specific care will vary according to the scenario, basic wilderness first-response steps can be applied in most medical emergencies, whether for yourself or when you're assisting someone else. It's a good idea to familiarize yourself with these steps so you can apply them in any given situation — particularly the stressful ones. Even if you're not a certified wilderness first responder or a wilderness emergency medical technician, don't worry; you can still come to someone's medical aid in style. In the end, just do your best. Your help, even if amateur, might make all the difference.

Assess your surroundings. Are you safe? Before rushing to help others, scan the area to make sure there aren't imminent threats that might add you to the victim count. No teetering rocks? No swarm of wasps? No signs of avalanche danger? Great, go help out.

Speak in a calm, comforting tone. If the coast is clear, approach the individual and ask if you can help.

Observe the scene. Does the person look ill or injured? What may have caused the illness or injury? This information may help you decide what to do next.

Use gloves. If they're available, put on some gloves before touching the person (because of bodily fluids).

Check the person's responsiveness. Ask them questions to check their alertness. Ask what their name is, what day it is and what happened.

Administer any immediate first aid. Prioritize the most serious injury or condition. That bandage isn't going to help much in the long run if the unconscious person isn't resuscitated.

Call for emergency help. If the situation is critical, or if the person can't transport themself out of the wilderness even with your assistance, call 911 if you're within cell range, or activate the SOS button on your satellite emergency device (see page 14).

Stay with the person. Until the situation resolves or help arrives, keep them comfortable.

1
BEFORE YOU GO

n advance of any outdoor adventure, do your homework because it could mean the difference between a fun and memorable trip or a dangerous and miserable one. The old saying "Prepare for the worst, hope for the best" is an apt one when it comes to venturing into nature. Take the following steps so everyone returns home safe and sound.

Assess your limits. How experienced is every person in your group? Does anyone need to take an avalanche course, a whitewater safety course or other classes that will prepare them for emergency scenarios? Is it worth hiring a guide or guide company, particularly if your activity requires specialized skills, like mountaineering, rafting or rock climbing? What's the medical status for each person in your group (allergies, illnesses, critical medications like insulin)? Check with your doctor if you have concerns about your own physical health.

Check the forecast. If the weather doesn't look optimal, consider rescheduling. Certain weather can lead to hazardous scenarios, such as flash floods, lightning storms, dangerous surf swells or avalanches. Knowing the weather beforehand can also help you pack — like knowing how many layers you may need and what kinds of supplies might be useful.

Pack appropriate gear. When considering what to bring, note the season, weather and planned activities. If you need to carry all your gear, weight and space will be important considerations. Make sure each person in the group knows what to pack and has all the gear they need to adventure safely.

Pack the right amount of water and food. Will water be available where you're planning to camp? Do you need to bring a water filtration or purification system? Does your activity allow you to bring perishable food (in a cooler, for example), or should you limit yourself to nonperishable, lightweight items?

EMERGENCY RESPONSE DEVICE

If you plan to adventure outside of cell range, it's a good idea to invest in a satellite emergency device. When you press the SOS button on these devices, they use satellites to determine your GPS location, then send that information to the appropriate response team. Usually, you'll need to pay a subscription fee for the time you plan on using the device. Be sure to store the device in an easy-to-reach location — holster it to your waist, for example — so you're not digging to the bottom of your backpack during an emergency.

Decide how many calories you'll need to consume to maintain steady energy levels and pack accordingly. Some healthy foods to pack that are lightweight and nutrient-dense include trail mix; nut-based granola or energy bars; dried or freeze-dried fruits and veggies; whole fruit that doesn't require refrigeration, such as apples, oranges and bananas; sandwiches that don't require refrigeration, such as peanut butter and jelly, and whole-grain bagels.

Do the math. How long will the drive take? How many miles do you need to bike on the first day? What class are the rapids you're planning to paddle? When does the sun rise and set? How many miles per hour do the people in your party hike? Doing some math ahead of time will help you arrive at destinations before dark, avoid sketchy scenarios and ensure that the scheduled mileage and activities will be manageable for all parties.

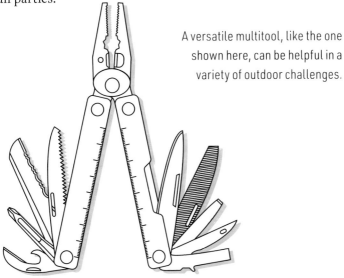

A versatile multitool, like the one shown here, can be helpful in a variety of outdoor challenges.

Do your research. What are the regulations, restrictions, permits, passes and fees for your destination? What wildlife do you need to prepare for (bears, snakes or mosquitoes)? Are the trails clear of fallen trees and branches? Are any roads or bridges washed out? Call the nearest ranger station ahead of time to get the scoop. Alternatively, check trip reports online. Trail and road conditions are often noted and dated by kind folks who want to make sure everyone has a great time.

Study those maps. Don't leave home without a map. While map apps on phones are handy, phones lose their charge, and chargers run out of battery. Bring a physical map as backup and plan your route before leaving home.

Come up with a Plan B. If someone gets injured on your long backpacking trip and you're 40 miles from the trailhead, what's your emergency response plan? Before leaving home, check your maps for possible exit strategies. If weather thwarts your plans, what other activities might you be able to do? Though it might be disappointing to alter your objectives, better safe than sorry.

Check in at the ranger station. If you're in a local, state or national park, let the local ranger station know your plans.

TRAVEL AND IMMUNIZATIONS

If your doctor asked you the date of your last tetanus shot, would you know the answer? A cut, laceration or other wound — even a minor one — can lead to a tetanus infection, so it's a good idea to stay up to date on your tetanus immunizations. After the initial tetanus series, booster shots are recommended every 10 years. If your most recent booster was more than five years ago, you may opt to get a tetanus shot after sustaining a deep or dirty wound.

If you're traveling out of the country, check the Centers for Disease Control website for a complete list of recommended vaccines and medicines for the country you plan to visit: *www.cdc.gov/travel*. If you've had any kind of surgery, particularly eye surgery, see a physician before traveling.

FIRST-AID KIT PACKING LIST

What and how much you pack in a first-aid kit will depend on the length of the trip, the number of people in your party, the types of activities you're doing and the weather forecast. It will also depend on how much packing space those activities allow for.

GIVE YOUR KIT A CHECKUP

+ Check your first-aid kits regularly to be sure the flashlight batteries work and to replace supplies that are expired or used up.
+ Consider taking a first-aid course through the American Red Cross. Contact your local chapter for information.
+ Prepare children for medical emergencies in ways that are age-appropriate. The American Red Cross offers a number of helpful resources, including classes designed to help children understand and use first-aid techniques.

FIRST-AID KIT PACKING LIST

BASIC SUPPLIES

+ First-aid manual
+ Adhesive tape
+ Elastic wrap bandages
+ Bandage strips and "butterfly" bandages, assorted sizes
+ Super glue
+ Rubber tourniquet or 16 French catheter
+ Nonstick sterile bandages of assorted sizes and gauze
+ Eye shield or pad
+ Triangular bandage that may be used as a sling
+ Aluminum finger splint
+ Instant cold packs
+ Cotton balls and cotton-tipped swabs
+ Disposable nonlatex examination gloves
+ Duct tape
+ Petroleum jelly or other lubricant
+ Safety pins, assorted sizes
+ Scissors and tweezers
+ Hand sanitizer
+ Antibiotic ointment
+ Antiseptic solution and towelettes
+ Eyewash solution
+ Thermometer
+ Turkey baster or other bulb suction device for flushing wounds
+ Sterile saline for irrigation, flushing
+ Breathing barrier (surgical mask)
+ Syringe, medicine cup or spoon
+ Hydrogen peroxide
+ Waterproof container to hold supplies
+ Moleskin pads
+ Insect repellent
+ Insect sting relief
+ Sunscreen

MEDICATIONS

+ Aloe vera gel
+ Calamine lotion
+ Anti-diarrhea medication
+ Laxatives
+ Antacids
+ Antihistamines, such as diphenhydramine (Benadryl, others)
+ Hydrocortisone cream
+ Triple antibiotic ointment
+ Aspirin
+ Cough and cold medications
+ Personal medications
+ Auto-injector of epinephrine, if prescribed
+ Pain relievers, such as acetaminophen (Tylenol, others) or ibuprofen (Advil, Motrin IB, others)

EMERGENCY ITEMS

+ Small, waterproof flashlight or headlamp and extra batteries
+ Waterproof matches
+ Small notepad and waterproof writing instrument
+ Emergency space blanket
+ Cellphone with solar charger
+ Iodine tablets or chlorine, for water purification
+ Oral thermometer
+ Emergency phone numbers, including contact information for your primary care provider, local emergency services, emergency road service providers, and the poison help line

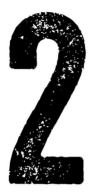

2

BLISTERS, BRUISES AND CUTS

listers, bruises and cuts are considered minor injuries. But anyone who's tried to hike after their heel puffed up into one giant blister may beg to differ. Have you ever banged your shin on a rock while scrambling over scree? Have you scraped your skin in a way that leaves it embedded with debris? These "minor" injuries can make babies out of the bravest of us and can become infected if not treated properly. Learning how to clean and bandage wounds will help promote their healing, prevent infection and reduce scarring.

BLISTERS

Blisters on your feet can turn the simple act of walking into a Herculean task. They can also form on your hands during activities like kayaking, canoeing, rock climbing and cycling.

No matter the sport, blisters are one of the most common wounds that occur in the outdoors. They're caused by the variables of pressure, heat, moisture, friction and burns. When skin rubs against the inside of a shoe, for example, blisters can form.

If a blister isn't too painful, try to keep it intact. Unbroken skin over a blister may provide a natural barrier to bacteria and decreases the risk of infection. Cover it with a bandage or moleskin. Moleskin is a durable fabric that can help protect blisters in high-friction areas. Cut a piece of moleskin slightly less than an inch larger than your blister. Fold the nonadhesive sides together and cut a half-circle that's about half the size of your blister. When you unfold it, you should have a hole in the middle about the size of your blister. Apply the donut-shaped pad over the blister, aligning your blister with the hole you made. Then cover the blister and moleskin with gauze.

Don't puncture a blister unless its location or the pain level prevents you from walking or using your hands. To relieve blister-related pain, drain the fluid while leaving the overlying skin intact (see Treatment » Blisters). If you're diabetic, have poor circulation or are predisposed to infections, be especially careful to prevent infection.

BLISTER PREVENTION

If you're blister-prone or simply trying an activity for the first time, it's worth taking some preventive measures.

+   **Wear appropriate gloves or socks.** Make sure they fit properly. Avoid cotton socks and opt for a moisture-wicking fabric. Before you go, test out various socks, shoes and insoles designed specifically to help reduce blistering.
+   **Add some powder.** Dust the inside of your socks with foot powder.

+ **Wear well-fitted shoes.** When buying new shoes:
  - » Shop later in the day, when your feet are typically more swollen.
  - » Wear the same socks you'll wear during your planned activity.
  - » Measure both feet and try on both shoes. If your feet differ in size, buy the larger size.
  - » Go for flexible but supportive shoes with cushioned insoles.
  - » Be sure you can comfortably wiggle your toes.
+ **Tape blister-prone spots.** If you experience recurring blisters in particular places, wrap the areas with tape (athletic tape works well, but duct tape is a decent backup).
+ **Add some padding.** Moleskin or gel-filled blister bandages can be used as preventive blister treatment.
+ **Tend to any hot spots right away.** Apply tape, padded blister bandages or moleskin over hot spots, which are areas where you can feel blisters beginning to form.
+ **Change into dry socks.** If your socks get too sweaty or soaked from a creek crossing, put on a fresh pair.

TREATMENT » BLISTERS

1. **Wash up.** Lather and rinse your hands and the blister with soap and water.
2. **Clean the site.** Swab the blister with an antiseptic wipe.
3. **Prepare a needle.** Sterilize a clean, sharp needle by wiping it with an antiseptic wipe or rubbing

PAGE 24

alcohol, or hold its pointed end in a flame for several seconds until the needle begins to turn red. Wipe off black carbon deposits with a sterile gauze pad and let the needle cool before inserting it.

4. **Use the needle to prick the blister.** Aim for several spots near the blister's edge. Let the fluid drain, but leave the overlying skin in place.

5. **Apply an ointment.** Apply an antibiotic ointment or petroleum jelly to the blister and cover it with a nonstick bandage or gauze pad.

6. **Aid the healing process.** After several days, cut away all the dead skin using tweezers and scissors sterilized with an antiseptic wipe. Apply more ointment and a bandage.

7. **Monitor for infection.** When you return home, call your doctor if you see signs of infection (pus, redness or discoloration, increasing pain or warm skin).

Needle method for draining a blister.
Using a sterilized needle, puncture the blister in several spots near the blister's edge. Let the fluid drain, but leave the skin in place.

BRUISES

A common cause of bruising is clumsiness, and nature doesn't help with all its tripping hazards. A bruise forms when blood vessels under the skin break. The trapped blood creates a bruise that's black, purple or blue, then changes color as it heals.

If your skin isn't broken, you don't need a bandage. You can, however, promote bruise healing with some simple techniques.

TREATMENT » BRUISES

1. **Elevate.** Raise the bruised area above heart level.
2. **Ice.** Apply an ice pack wrapped in a thin towel. Leave it in place for 20 minutes. Repeat several times for a day or two after the injury.
3. **Compress.** If the bruised area is swelling, put an elastic bandage around it, but not too tight.
4. **Take medication.** Consider an over-the-counter (nonprescription) pain reliever if needed.

SEEK MEDICAL ATTENTION IF YOU:

+ Have painful swelling in the bruised area.
+ Are still experiencing pain three days after a seemingly minor injury.
+ Notice a lump form over the bruise.

If a bruise is severe or worsening, you may need to abandon your trip and get medical help.

CUTS

Let's face it, nature is sharp. Not only do you have to watch out for sticks, thorns, cactus spines, rock edges and claws, but there are also other dangers about. Glissade down a snow slope with a little too much enthusiasm and you might scrape exposed skin.

Seek medical help for a wound that is deep, is gaping, or has fat or muscle protruding from it. If your wound is deep or dirty and your last tetanus shot was more than five years ago, ask your doctor if you need a booster shot.

Minor cuts and scrapes usually don't require a trip to the emergency department. Yet proper care is essential to avoid complications. The guidelines below can help you care for minor cuts and scrapes.

TREATMENT » MINOR CUTS AND SCRAPES

1. **Wash your hands.** This helps avoid infection.
2. **Stop the bleeding.** Minor cuts and scrapes usually stop bleeding on their own. If needed, apply gentle pressure with a clean cloth or bandage and elevate the wound until bleeding stops. Hold the pressure continuously for 20 to 30 minutes. Don't keep checking to see if the bleeding has stopped, as this may damage the fresh clot that's forming.
3. **Clean the wound.** After the bleeding has stopped, gently rinse the wound with water.

Keeping the wound under running tap water will reduce the risk of infection. Wash around the wound with soap. But don't get soap in the wound. And don't use hydrogen peroxide or iodine, which can be irritating. Remove any dirt or debris with tweezers cleaned with alcohol. Seek medical help if you can't remove all debris.

4. **Apply an antibiotic.** After cleaning the wound, apply a thin layer of an antibiotic ointment or petroleum jelly to keep the surface moist and to help prevent scarring. Certain ingredients in some ointments can cause a mild rash in some people. If a rash appears, stop using the ointment.

5. **Cover the wound.** Apply a bandage, rolled gauze or gauze held in place with paper tape. Covering the wound keeps it clean. If the injury is just a minor scrape or scratch, leave it uncovered.

6. **Change the dressing.** Do this at least once a day or whenever the bandage becomes wet or dirty.

7. **Get a tetanus shot.** You may need a tetanus shot if you haven't had one in the past five years and the wound is deep or dirty.

8. **Watch for signs of infection.** See a doctor if you see signs of infection on the skin or near the wound, such as redness or discoloration, increasing pain, drainage, warmth or swelling.

3
STINGS AND BITES

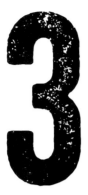

Looking to avoid unwelcome surprises? Shake out those shoes and sleeping bags. Outdoor adventure means getting up close and personal with buzzing, crawling, rattling risks that can, at a minimum, be an unbearable bother. Even a nuisance as seemingly minor as a mosquito bite can bring the toughest people to their knees. At their worst, bites and stings can pose threats of infection, allergic reactions or life-threatening reactions to poison. So, watch where you step and swim. Shield yourself with repellent and protective clothing. Maintain a respectful distance from wildlife. Before traveling, research the common insects, spiders, snakes and animals that might pose risks in that area. Most important, stay calm and treat any bite or sting with the appropriate first-aid response.

Immediate medical care is recommended for anyone who has symptoms of a severe reaction. If you have cell service, while waiting for medical care to arrive, call Poison Control at 1-800-222-1222. It offers free, confidential care 24 hours a day.

STINGS

Venom from certain insects, scorpions or sea organisms can pack a potent sting. Usually, stings are temporarily uncomfortable. Sometimes, though, more serious symptoms develop that require medical attention.

INSECT STINGS

Most insect stings are mild and can be managed without emergency medical intervention. They might cause itching, swelling, redness or discoloration and burning that are limited to the area of the sting and go away in a day or two. However, your entire body can be affected if the venom is potent or if you're hypersensitive to the toxins. Stings from bees, yellow jackets, wasps, hornets and fire ants might cause a severe allergic reaction (anaphylaxis).

All insect stings should be treated promptly to minimize risks of infection, an allergic reaction or other complications.

TREATMENT » MILD REACTIONS TO INSECT STINGS

1. **Move.** Move to a safe area to avoid more stings.
2. **Remove any stingers.** You can do this by wiping gauze or a straight-edged object, like the blunt side of a knife on a multitool, over the sting site. Gently wash the area with soap and water.

3. **Reduce swelling.** Apply a cloth dampened with cold water or filled with ice to the area of the bite or sting for 10 to 20 minutes.
4. **Elevate.** If the injury is on an arm or leg, raise it.
5. **Alleviate symptoms.** Apply calamine lotion, a paste of baking soda and water, or 0.5% or 1% hydrocortisone cream to the affected area. Do this up to four times a day until your symptoms go away. You also can take an oral anti-itch medicine (antihistamine). Be aware that some antihistamines can make you drowsy.
6. **Relieve pain.** Take a nonprescription pain reliever if needed.

Remove an insect stinger by scraping a straight-edged object, like the blunt edge of a knife on a multitool, over the area.

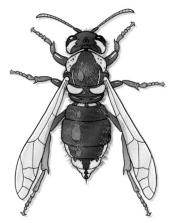

HONEYBEE
Fuzzy, pollen-gathering.

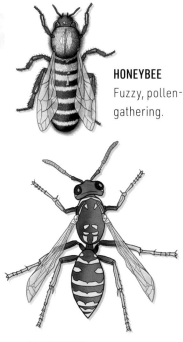

WHITE-FACED (BALD-FACED) HORNET
Mostly black and white.

PAPER WASP
Smaller than hornets, slender with smoky black wings.

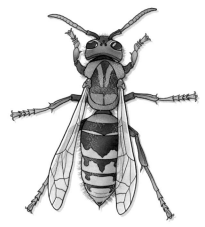

YELLOW (EUROPEAN) HORNET
Dotted banding.

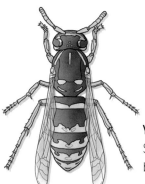

YELLOWJACKET
Smaller than hornets, yellow with black dots and stripes across abdomen.

SCORPION STINGS

Scorpion stings are painful but rarely life-threatening. In the United States, the bark scorpion, found mainly in the desert Southwest, is the only scorpion species with venom potent enough to cause severe symptoms. As with other stinging insects, such as bees and wasps, it's possible for people who've previously been stung by scorpions to have allergic reactions with subsequent stings. Reactions to subsequent stings are sometimes still severe enough to cause a serious reaction (anaphylaxis).

Signs and symptoms at the site of a scorpion sting may include pain, numbness and tingling, slight swelling and warmth. Children under the age of 6 and older adults are most at risk of serious complications. Seek immediate medical care for a child stung by a scorpion, or if an adult begins to experience severe symptoms after a scorpion sting.

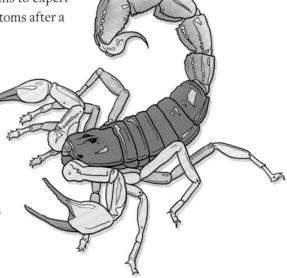

BARK SCORPION
The bark scorpion is venomous, but only stings if it feels threatened. Best to leave it alone.

+ Difficulty breathing
+ Muscle twitching or thrashing
+ Drooling
+ Sweating
+ Nausea and vomiting
+ High blood pressure
+ Accelerated heart rate
+ Restlessness or excitability, or inconsolable crying in children

Most scorpion stings don't need medical treatment. But if symptoms are severe, you may need prompt medical attention. Scorpion antivenom may be given to children to prevent the progression of symptoms. Adults with severe symptoms also may receive antivenom. Make sure tetanus vaccines are up to date. If a scorpion stings you or your child, follow basic first aid. Healthy adults may not need further treatment. First aid can help keep children safe until they see a doctor.

TREATMENT » SCORPION STINGS

1. **Wash.** Clean the site with mild soap and water.
2. **Ice it.** Apply a cool compress to the affected area.
3. **Fast.** Don't consume food or liquids if you're having difficulty swallowing.
4. **Take medication.** Take an over-the-counter pain reliever as needed to help ease discomfort.

Jellyfish stings are fairly common among people swimming, wading or diving in oceans. The long tentacles trailing from the jellyfish can inject venom from thousands of microscopic barbed stingers. Jellyfish that have washed up on a beach may still release venomous stingers if touched. Most often, jellyfish stings cause instant pain and welts or tracks on the skin — a "print" of the tentacles' contact with the skin. Other symptoms include itchiness, swelling, and throbbing pain that radiates up a leg or an arm. The stings usually get better over a few days or weeks with home treatment.

Some stings may cause more widespread illness. In rare cases the stings can be life-threatening. Reactions may appear rapidly or over several hours after the sting. The severity of a reaction depends on:

+ The type and size of the jellyfish.
+ The age, size and health of the person affected.
+ How long the person was exposed to the stingers.
+ How much of the skin is affected.

Types of jellyfish

Most types of jellyfish are fairly harmless to humans. Others can cause severe pain

BOX JELLYFISH

and a full-body (systemic) reaction. These jellyfish cause more serious problems:

+ **Box jellyfish.** This type can cause intense pain and, rarely, life-threatening reactions. The more dangerous species of box jellyfish are located in the warm waters of the Pacific and Indian oceans.

+ **Portuguese man-of-war.** Also called bluebottle jellyfish, Portuguese man-of-war jellyfish live mostly in warmer seas. This type has a blue or purplish gas-filled bubble that keeps it afloat.

+ **Sea nettle.** It's common in both warm and cool seawaters.

+ **Lion's mane jellyfish.** These are the world's largest jellyfish, with a body diameter of more than 3 feet. They're most common in cooler, northern regions of the Pacific and Atlantic oceans.

SIGNS AND SYMPTOMS »
JELLYFISH STINGS, SEVERE REACTION

+ Stomach pain, nausea and vomiting
+ Headache
+ Muscle pain or spasms
+ Faintness, dizziness or confusion
+ Difficulty breathing
+ Heart problems

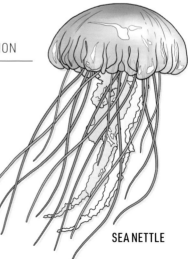

SEA NETTLE

1. **Get out of the water.**
Pain and cramps can
become disabling, increasing
the risk of drowning.

2. **Remove any tentacles.**
Carefully pluck visible tentacles
with fine tweezers.

3. **Soak the sting site.** Soak the skin
in water that's hot — like a hot
shower — but not boiling. Keep
the affected skin immersed in hot
water until the pain eases, which
may be 20 to 45 minutes.

**PORTUGUESE
MAN-OF-WAR**

4. **Apply ointment.** Apply 0.5% to 1%
hydrocortisone cream or ointment
twice a day to the affected skin.

5. **Assess the severity.** Severe
reactions, including collapse
and the need for CPR, can
occur from jellyfish stings.
A severe reaction to a box
jellyfish sting may be treated
with antivenom medication.
All stings on or near the eye
should be seen by a doctor.

LION'S MANE JELLYFISH

PAGE 38

Steps to avoid

These myths surrounding the treatment of jellyfish stings don't work and should be avoided:

+ Scraping out stingers
+ Rinsing with human urine
+ Rinsing with cold, fresh water
+ Applying meat tenderizer
+ Applying alcohol, ethanol or ammonia
+ Rubbing with a towel
+ Applying pressure bandages

ANAPHYLACTIC SHOCK

A life-threatening allergic reaction (anaphylaxis) can cause shock, a sudden drop in blood pressure and trouble breathing. In people who have a severe allergy, anaphylaxis can occur minutes after exposure to a specific allergy-causing substance (allergen). In some cases, there may be a delayed reaction, or anaphylaxis may occur without an obvious trigger.

SIGNS AND SYMPTOMS » ANAPHYLACTIC SHOCK

+ Skin reactions, including hives, itching, and skin that becomes flushed or changes color
+ Swelling of the face, eyes, lips or throat
+ A weak and rapid pulse

- Narrowing of the airways, leading to wheezing and trouble breathing or swallowing
- Nausea, vomiting or diarrhea
- Dizziness, fainting or unconsciousness

TREATMENT » ANAPHYLACTIC SHOCK

If you're with someone experiencing an allergic reaction with signs of anaphylaxis, don't wait to see if the symptoms start to get better:

1. Immediately call 911 if you're within cell range or activate the SOS button on an emergency device.
2. Ask if the person is carrying an epinephrine autoinjector (EpiPen, Auvi-Q, others) to treat an allergic attack.
3. If the person needs to use an autoinjector, ask whether you should help inject the medication. This is usually done by pressing the autoinjector against the person's thigh.
4. Have the person lie face up and be still.
5. Loosen tight clothing and cover the person with a blanket. Don't give the person anything to drink.
6. If there's vomiting or bleeding from the mouth, turn the person onto their side to prevent choking.
7. If there are no signs of breathing, coughing or movement, begin CPR (see page 135).
8. Get emergency treatment even if symptoms start to improve. After anaphylaxis, it's possible for symptoms to recur.

 PAGE 40

40

In severe cases, untreated anaphylaxis can lead to death within half an hour.

An antihistamine pill, such as diphenhydramine (Benadryl), isn't enough to treat anaphylaxis. These medications can help relieve allergy symptoms, but they work too slowly in a severe reaction. Insect stings from bees, yellowjackets, wasps, hornets and fire ants are common anaphylaxis triggers.

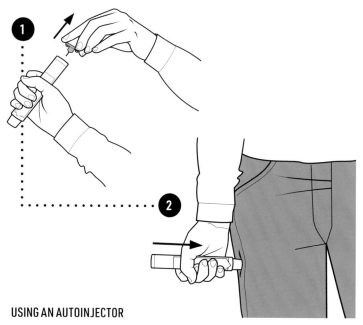

USING AN AUTOINJECTOR

Follow product instructions. The tip of the device should be held at a right angle to the middle of the front thigh or middle of the outer thigh. Swing and push the autoinjector firmly into the thigh until it "clicks." Hold it in place to a count of three.

INSECT BITES

A minor insect bite can produce a bump on the skin that might itch or cause discomfort for a few hours to a few days. The bites of mosquitoes, flies, ants and chiggers often follow this course. However, insects like mosquitos and ticks can carry disease, so it's always a good idea to take precautions to prevent bites.

Such measures can include spraying insect repellent, which should be applied on top of sunscreen. Insect repellent should contain 25% to 30% DEET or 15% or more of picaridin. Keep track of when you need to reapply: 10% DEET is effective for two hours, 20% DEET is effective for about five hours and 20% picaridin is effective for 10 hours. Insect-repellent clothing can also help, though it doesn't protect exposed skin. Combining the two — wearing insect-repellent clothing and spraying insect repellent on exposed skin — offers thorough protection.

MOSQUITOES AND OTHERS

Not only is the mosquito's high-pitched whine a notorious nuisance in the outdoors, but mosquito bites can cause severe illnesses if the insects carry certain viruses or parasites. Infected mosquitoes can spread West Nile virus, Zika virus, and the viruses that cause malaria and yellow fever.

Bites from horseflies, deer flies, black flies, sand flies, midges and chiggers may cause localized itchiness or irritation. Flies can also carry diseases such as typhoid fever, dysentery and cholera. Therefore, prevention of insect bites is key.

+ **Avoid and exclude insects.** Limit exposure to insects by repairing tears in the screens on camping gear, using mosquito netting while sleeping outdoors, and using unscented self-care products.

+ **Use insect repellent when insects are active.** The most effective insect repellents in the United States include one of these active ingredients:

  » DEET
  » Picaridin, also called icaridin
  » Oil of lemon or eucalyptus
  » IR3535
  » Para-menthane-diol (PMD)
  » 2-Undecanone

  These ingredients temporarily repel mosquitoes and ticks. If you're using a spray repellent, apply it outdoors and away from food. If you're also using sunscreen, put it on first, about 20 minutes before applying insect repellent.

  » **Read the label before applying.** Used according to package directions, these products are generally safe for children and adults, with a few exceptions:

    • Don't use DEET-containing products on infants younger than 2 months.
    • Don't use icaridin on infants younger than 6 months.
    • Don't use PMD on children younger than 3 years.
    • Don't let young children get insect repellent on their hands, as they might get it in their mouths.

- Don't apply repellent near the eyes and mouth.
- Don't apply repellent, especially DEET, under clothing.
- Don't apply insect repellent over sunburns, wounds, cuts or rashes.
- When the risk of mosquito bites has passed, wash repellent off the skin with soap and water.

+ **Treat clothing and outdoor gear.** Permethrin is an insecticide and insect repellent used for added protection. This product is made to use on clothing and outdoor gear, not on the skin. Clothing sprayed with permethrin can offer protection for two washings and up to two weeks. Check the product label for instructions.

+ **Use protective clothing and gear.** Weather permitting, wear a hat, long-sleeved shirts and long pants.

+ **Take preventive medicine.** Get vaccinations or take preventive medicine as prescribed or suggested by a medical professional. If you tend to have large or severe reactions to mosquito bites, you may want to take a nondrowsy, nonprescription antihistamine when you know you'll be exposed to mosquitoes.

SIGNS AND SYMPTOMS » MOSQUITO BITES

+ An itchy, inflamed bump that forms a few minutes after the bite
+ A painful spot that looks like a hive and forms within 24 hours after a bite
+ Small blisters

A more severe reaction can cause:

+ A large, swollen, inflamed area
+ A hive-like rash
+ Swelling around the eyes

Seek medical assistance if the mosquito bites seem to occur with warning signs of a serious condition, such as a high fever, severe headache, body aches and indications of infection.

TREATMENT » MOSQUITO BITES

Most mosquito bites stop itching and heal on their own in a few days. These self-care tips may make you more comfortable.

1. **Apply a lotion, cream or paste.** Avoid scratching itchy bites, as this can lead to infection. It may help to apply calamine lotion or a nonprescription antihistamine cream or corticosteroid cream. Or try dabbing the bite with a paste made of baking soda and water. Reapply the cream or the paste three times a day until the itch is gone.

2. **Rub with an ice cube.** Try soothing an itchy bite by rubbing it with an ice cube for 30 seconds.

3. **Apply pressure.** Another way to soothe an itchy bite is by applying pressure for 10 seconds.

4. **Take an oral antihistamine.** For stronger reactions, try taking a nonprescription antihistamine that doesn't cause sleepiness.

TICK BITES

Some ticks carry infections that can be transmitted to humans by a bite. American dog ticks and Rocky Mountain wood ticks can carry Rocky Mountain spotted fever. Deer ticks — which are much smaller than wood ticks — can carry Lyme disease and anaplasmosis. In general, to transmit Lyme disease a tick needs to be attached to a person's skin for at least 36 hours. Other infections can be transferred in a few hours or even a few minutes.

Rocky Mountain spotted fever can produce chills and fever, severe headaches, widespread aches, restlessness and a red rash occurring between days two and six of the onset of fever. Lyme disease may produce symptoms of fatigue, headache and muscle and joint pain, along with a characteristic nonpainful rash, often with a target or bull's-eye appearance. Anaplasmosis may cause fever, malaise, headache and general body aches.

BLACK-LEGGED (DEER) TICK

The black-legged tick, also known as a deer tick, is mainly located in the eastern half and north-central region of the U.S. It's responsible for spreading several tick-borne illnesses including Lyme disease.

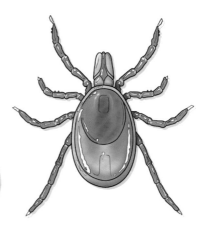

ACTUAL SIZE
(3-10 mm)

MAYO CLINIC FIRST-AID GUIDE FOR OUTDOOR ADVENTURES

1. **Remove the tick promptly and carefully.** Use fine-tipped forceps or tweezers to grasp the tick as close to the skin as possible. Gently pull out the tick. Don't handle it with bare hands. And don't use petroleum jelly, fingernail polish or a hot match to remove it.

2. **Place the tick in a container or take a picture.** This can help identify what type it is and whether you may be at risk of a transmitted disease.

3. **Wash your hands and the bite site.** Use warm water and soap or rubbing alcohol.

4. **Monitor symptoms.** If you're able to remove the body of the tick, you've removed the risk of transmitting disease, even if part of the head or tiny mouth parts remain. The bite site can get infected. If you suspect an infection, which may include pain, a change in skin color and oozing from the site, seek medical care. Also seek care if you develop a fever, stiff neck, flu-like symptoms or a rash with a bull's-eye pattern.

TO REMOVE A TICK
Use tweezers to grab the tick as close to its head as possible. Slowly and steadily pull the tick away from the skin.

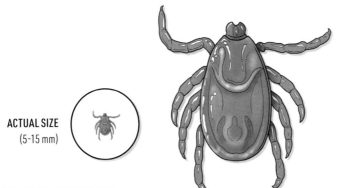

ACTUAL SIZE
(5-15 mm)

AMERICAN DOG (WOOD) TICK

The American dog tick, also known as a wood tick, is mainly located east of the U.S. Rocky Mountains and in some areas of the Pacific Coast. It's responsible for spreading Rocky Mountain spotted fever and a bacterial disease called tularemia.

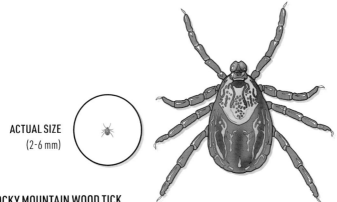

ACTUAL SIZE
(2-6 mm)

ROCKY MOUNTAIN WOOD TICK

The Rocky Mountain wood tick is mainly located in the U.S. Rocky Mountain states and Southwestern Canada. It's responsible for spreading Colorado tick fever, Rocky Mountain spotted fever and the bacterial disease tularemia.

VENOMOUS SPIDER BITES

Only a few spiders are dangerous to humans. Two found in the contiguous United States and more commonly in the Southern states are the black widow and brown recluse. Both types of spiders prefer warm and dark, dry places where flies are plentiful, such as woodpiles and areas where debris has accumulated. Spiders usually aren't aggressive and most bites occur because a spider is trapped or unintentionally touched.

Seek medical care right away if:

+ You've been bitten by a black widow or brown recluse spider.
+ You're unsure whether the bite was from a dangerous spider.
+ You have severe pain, stomach cramping or a growing wound at the bite site.
+ You're having problems breathing or swallowing.
+ The area of inflamed skin is spreading or has streaks.

BLACK WIDOW SPIDER

Black widow spiders are found throughout North America but are most common in the Southern and Western areas of the United States. They're identified by a pattern of red markings on the underside of their abdomen. They're usually found in undisturbed areas but may also be found in outdoor toilets.

Black widow spiders build webs between objects, and bites usually occur when humans come into direct contact with these webs. A bite from a black widow can be distinguished from other insect bites by the two puncture marks the spider makes in the skin. Its venom produces pain at the site of the bite and then spreads to the chest, abdomen or the entire body.

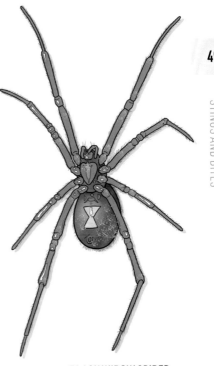

BLACK WIDOW SPIDER

SIGNS AND SYMPTOMS »
BLACK WIDOW SPIDER BITE

+ Inflamed skin, pain and swelling
+ Severe stomach pain or cramping
+ Nausea, vomiting, shaking or sweating

BROWN RECLUSE SPIDER

The brown recluse spider is most commonly found in the Midwestern and Southern states. It's brown in color with a characteristic dark violin-shaped (or fiddle-shaped) marking on its head. It has six equal-sized eyes (most spiders have eight eyes). Brown recluse spiders are usually found in secluded, dry, sheltered areas such as underneath logs, or in piles of rocks or leaves.

The brown recluse spider cannot bite humans without some form of counter pressure, for example, through unintentional contact that traps the spider against the skin. Bites may cause a stinging sensation with localized pain. A small white blister usually develops at the site of the bite. The venom of a brown recluse can cause a severe lesion by destroying skin tissue (skin necrosis), which requires attention from a medical professional.

SIGNS AND SYMPTOMS » BROWN RECLUSE SPIDER BITE

+ At first, a mild pain
+ Fever, chills and body aches
+ A sore with a blue or purple center and ring around it

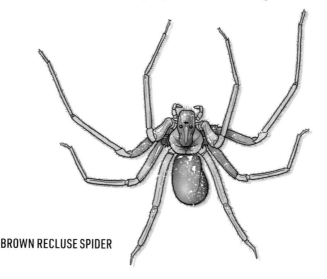

BROWN RECLUSE SPIDER

1. **Wash up and apply ointment.** Clean the wound with soap and water and apply an antibiotic cream three times a day to help prevent infection.
2. **Cool it.** Apply a cool cloth over the bite for 15 minutes every hour. Use a clean cloth dampened with water or filled with ice.
3. **Elevate.** If possible, elevate the affected area.
4. **Take medication.** Take a nonprescription pain reliever as needed for pain.
5. **Soothe the itch.** If the wound is itchy, an antihistamine cream or ointment or an oral antihistamine might help. Or use a steroid cream.
6. **Monitor signs and symptoms.** Seek immediate medical attention if they become severe.

VENOMOUS SNAKE BITES

Most snakes aren't dangerous to people. Only about 15% of snakes worldwide and 20% in the United States can inject poison when they bite. These snakes are called venomous.

TYPES OF VENOMOUS SNAKES

In North America, venomous snakes include the rattle-snake, coral snake, water moccasin, also called cottonmouth, and copperhead. Their bites can cause serious injuries and sometimes death.

Most venomous snakes in North America have eyes like slits and are called pit vipers. Their heads are triangle-shaped and they have fangs. One exception is the coral snake, which has a cigar-shaped head and round pupils. Nonvenomous snakes typically have rounded heads, round pupils and no fangs.

Rattlesnakes

Rattlesnakes are the largest venomous snake in the United States. Whether coiled or stretched out, they can quickly and accurately strike at a distance of one-third or more of their body length from any position. Rattlesnakes may use their rattle as a warning when they feel threatened, but they don't always rattle before biting.

Rattlesnakes live in many habitats, including in the mountains, prairies, deserts, and beaches throughout the United States.

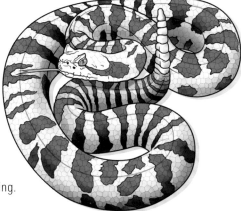

RATTLESNAKE
May use their rattle
as a warning but don't
always rattle before biting.

WATER MOCCASIN (COTTONMOUTH)
Adult's skin is dark tan,
brown, or nearly black, with
vague cross-bands. Juveniles
have bold brown or orange
cross-bands with a yellow tail.

COPPERHEAD
Varies in color from
reddish to golden tan
with hourglass-shaped
colored bands on the body.

CORAL SNAKE
Has bands of red,
yellow and black.
The red bands are
surrounded on both
sides by smaller yellow bands.

Water moccasins

Water moccasins, also called cottonmouths, have a whitish, cottony lining in their mouths. Adult cottonmouth snakes average 50 to 55 inches long. The adult snake's skin is dark tan, brown, or nearly black, with vague black or dark brown cross-bands. Juvenile snakes have a bold cross-banded pattern of brown or orange with a yellow tail. These snakes are often found in or around water in the Southeastern states.

Copperheads

Copperheads vary in color from reddish to golden tan. The colored bands on their bodies are typically hourglass-shaped. They have a deep facial pit between each eye and their nostril. Most adults are about 18 to 36 inches long. These snakes are not usually aggressive, but they will often freeze when approached and then strike in defense if threatened, contacted or interacted with. Copperheads are often found in forests, rocky areas, swamps, or near sources of water like rivers in the Eastern states, extending as far west as Texas.

Coral snakes

These snakes are sometimes confused with nonvenomous king snakes, which have similar colored bands, but arranged differently. Coral snakes tend to hide in leafy piles or burrow into the ground. They're commonly found in wooded, sandy or marshy areas of the Southern United States.

DRY BITES

Sometimes, a venomous snake can bite without injecting venom. This is called a dry bite. Typical symptoms of a nonvenomous snake bite are pain, injury and scratches at the site of the bite.

SIGNS AND SYMPTOMS » VENOMOUS SNAKE BITES

+ Severe pain and tenderness at the site of the bite
+ Swelling, bruising, bleeding or blistering around the site that may move all the way up the arm or leg
+ Nausea, vomiting or diarrhea
+ Labored breathing
+ Rapid heart rate, weak pulse, low blood pressure
+ Changes in vision
+ Numbness or tingling in the face or limbs
+ Muscle twitching
+ An odd taste in the mouth

TREATMENT » VENOMOUS SNAKE BITES

If a venomous snake bites you, immediately call 911 or activate the SOS button on an emergency device. If possible, take these steps while waiting for medical help:

1. Move far away from the snake.
2. Stay still and calm.
3. Remove any jewelry, watches or tight clothing on the affected limb before swelling starts.

PAGE 56

4. Sit or lie down so that the bite is in a neutral, comfortable position.
5. Clean the bite with soap and water.
6. Cover or wrap the affected area loosely with a clean, dry bandage.

Caution

+ Don't use a tourniquet or apply ice.
+ Don't cut the bite or try to remove the venom by squeezing or sucking the wound.
+ Don't drink caffeine or alcohol.
+ Don't take pain-relieving medication.
+ Don't try to catch or trap the snake, but try to remember its color so you can describe it.

ANIMAL AND HUMAN BITES

Animals don't have to be sick to be a risk to humans. The normal bacteria of some animals can cause serious infections in humans, and some animals can be carriers of disease. Though attacks by domestic animals are far more common than those by wildlife, any animal can attack if it feels threatened, is protecting its young or territory, or is injured or ill. Adventurers should exercise caution around wild animals, maintain a safe distance and address any scratches or bites right away.

Human bites can be just as dangerous as animal bites because of bacteria and viruses located in the human mouth.

Human bites that break the skin can become infected. If you cut your knuckles on another person's teeth that also is considered a human bite, as is a cut on the knuckles from your own teeth.

To care for a minor bite or claw wound, such as one that only breaks the skin, treat it as you would a minor wound (see page 26). To treat a deep wound, seek emergency medical care and follow steps to stop severe bleeding, if necessary (see page 75).

TREATMENT » ANIMAL & HUMAN BITES

1. **Stop the bleeding.** Apply pressure with a clean, dry cloth.
2. **Wash up.** Thoroughly clean the wound with soap and water.
3. **Apply a clean bandage.** Cover the affected area with a nonstick bandage.
4. **Get help.** See a doctor to prevent infection.

Seek prompt medical care if:

+ The wound is deep.
+ The skin is badly torn, crushed or bleeding significantly.
+ You notice increasing swelling, redness or discoloration, pain or oozing.
+ You have concerns about the risk of rabies.
+ You haven't had a tetanus shot in the past 10 years — or five years if the wound is deep or dirty.

RISK OF RABIES

Rabies is a deadly virus spread to people from the saliva of infected animals, usually through a bite. Animals most likely to transmit rabies in the United States include bats, coyotes, foxes, raccoons and skunks, but any mammal can spread the virus.

Once a person begins showing signs of rabies, the disease nearly always causes death. For this reason, if you've been in contact with any wildlife or unfamiliar animals, you should talk with a healthcare or public health professional to determine your risk for rabies or other illnesses.

RABIES IN BATS

Unlike other animals that carry rabies, many types of bats have very small teeth which may leave marks that disappear quickly. Bats are one of the most commonly reported rabid animals in the United States and are the leading cause of rabies deaths. If you know you've been bitten or scratched by a bat, or if you're unsure whether you've been bitten, wash the wound thoroughly with soap and water and seek medical attention immediately.

RABIES IN ANIMALS

You can't tell if an animal has rabies by just looking at it. However, animals with rabies may act strangely, may be aggressive and try to bite you or they may drool more than normal. (This is sometimes portrayed in movies as animals "foaming at the mouth.") But not all animals with rabies will be aggressive or drooling. Other animals may act timid or shy, move slowly and let you get close to them. That's not characteristic of the way wild animals usually act. Be careful.

SIGNS AND SYMPTOMS » RABIES IN ANIMALS

+ General sickness
+ Problems swallowing
+ Excessive drool or saliva
+ An animal that's overly aggressive
+ An animal that bites at imaginary objects (sometimes called "fly biting")
+ An animal that appears tamer than you would expect
+ An animal that's having trouble moving or may be paralyzed
+ A bat that's on the ground

TREATMENT » RABIES EXPOSURE

1. **Wash up.** Thoroughly clean the wound with soap and water.
2. **Get help.** Seek medical attention immediately. A series of shots is given to prevent the rabies virus from causing infection.

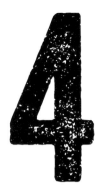

4

BURNS

tay alert while using that camp stove, and be careful not to pour boiling water or coffee on your hand. Always be cautious around the campfire. Protect your skin from the sun's ultraviolet (UV) rays. Know what to do if you're caught in a lightning storm while outdoors. Burns can come from a variety of sources in the wilderness, so it's important to practice proper safety and to learn how to treat burns if they do occur.

Burns are tissue damage from hot liquids, the sun, flames, chemicals, electricity, steam and other causes. Major burns need emergency medical help. Minor burns can usually be treated with first aid.

BURN CLASSIFICATIONS

To distinguish a minor burn from a serious burn, the first step is to determine the degree and the extent of damage to body tissues. The severity of your wound, based on depth, size, and location, will indicate the need for specialized care.

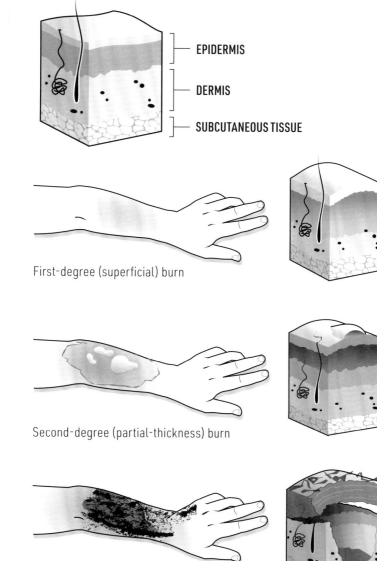

EPIDERMIS

DERMIS

SUBCUTANEOUS TISSUE

First-degree (superficial) burn

Second-degree (partial-thickness) burn

Third-degree (full-thickness) burn

FIRST-DEGREE BURN

Superficial burns affect only the outer layer of skin (epidermis), and the skin doesn't blister. These kinds of burns may cause redness or discoloration, swelling and pain.

SECOND-DEGREE BURN

This type of burn affects both the epidermis and the second layer of skin (dermis). It may cause swelling, weeping, and red, white or splotchy skin. Blisters develop, and pain can be intense. Deep second-degree burns can lead to scarring.

THIRD-DEGREE BURN

These burns involve all of the layers of skin — and sometimes deeper tissue, such as fat or muscle — and they cause permanent tissue damage. Blisters don't develop. Because nerve damage is substantial, there's minimal pain or none at all. These burns need emergency care and often require surgical intervention.

TREATMENT » MINOR BURNS

1. **Cool the burn.** Hold the area under cool (not cold) running water for about 10 minutes. If this isn't possible, or if the burn is on the face, apply a cool, wet cloth until the pain eases.

PAGE 64

2. **Remove rings, watches or other tight items from the burned area.** Try to do this quickly and gently, before the area swells.

3. **Don't break blisters.** Blisters help protect against infection. If a blister does break, gently clean the area with water and apply an antibiotic ointment.

4. **Apply lotion.** After the burn is cooled, apply a lotion, such as one with aloe vera or cocoa butter. This helps prevent drying and provides relief.

5. **Bandage the burn.** Cover the burn with a clean bandage. Wrap it loosely to avoid putting pressure on burned skin. Bandaging keeps air off the area, reduces pain and protects blistered skin.

6. **If needed, take a nonprescription pain reliever.** These include ibuprofen (Advil, Motrin IB, others) or acetaminophen (Tylenol, others).

SIGNS AND SYMPTOMS » MAJOR BURNS

+ May be deep, involving all layers of the skin
+ May cause the skin to be dry and leathery
+ May appear charred or have patches of waxy white, brown or black
+ Are larger than 3 inches in diameter
+ Cover the hands, feet, face, groin, buttocks or a major joint, or encircle an arm or leg
+ Are accompanied by smoke inhalation
+ Begin swelling very quickly

Both electrical burns, including those caused by lightning, and major chemical burns need emergency medical care. A minor burn might need emergency care if it affects the eyes, mouth, hands or genital areas. Babies and older adults might need emergency care for minor burns as well.

TREATMENT » MAJOR BURNS

Until emergency help arrives:

1. **Protect the burned person from further harm.** If you can do so safely, make sure the person you're helping is not in contact with the source of the burn.

2. **Don't try to remove clothing stuck in the burn.**

3. **Remove jewelry, belts and other tight items, especially from the burned area.** Burned areas swell quickly.

4. **Cover the burn.** Loosely cover the area with gauze or a clean cloth.

5. **Raise the burned area.** Lift the wound above heart level if possible.

6. **Watch for signs of shock.** Signs and symptoms include cool, clammy skin, weak pulse and shallow breathing. For information on treating shock, see page 177.

7. **Make certain that the person burned is breathing.** If needed, begin rescue breathing if you know how.

SUNBURN

If you've been sunburned, you'll notice signs and symptoms within a few hours of being out in the sun. The affected skin may be painful, inflamed and hot to the touch. Blisters might develop. You also may experience headache, fever or nausea. Seek immediate medical care if you're sunburned and experience:

+ A fever greater than 103 F with vomiting.
+ Confusion or passing out.
+ An infection over the sunburned area.
+ Dehydration.

TREATMENT » SUNBURN

To help relieve sunburn discomfort:

1. **Take a pain reliever.** Take ibuprofen (Advil, Motrin IB, others) or acetaminophen (Tylenol, others).
2. **Cool the skin.** Apply to sunburned skin a clean towel dampened with cool tap water. Or take a cool bath, if possible. Add about 2 ounces of baking soda to the tub. Cool the skin for about 10 minutes several times a day.
3. **Apply a moisturizer, lotion or gel.** Aloe vera lotion or gel or calamine lotion can be soothing. Try cooling the product in the refrigerator before applying. Avoid products that contain alcohol.
4. **Apply a medicated cream.** For mild to moderate sunburn, apply nonprescription 1%

hydrocortisone cream to the affected area three times a day for three days. Try cooling the product before applying.

5. **Drink extra water.** This helps prevent dehydration.

6. **Leave blisters alone.** An intact blister can help the skin heal. If a blister does break, trim off the dead skin with clean, small scissors. Gently clean the area with mild soap and water. Then apply an antibiotic ointment to the wound and cover it with a nonstick bandage (see page 23).

7. **Don't re-burn.** Protect yourself from further sun exposure while your skin heals from the sunburn.

8. **Care for your eyes.** Treat sunburned eyes by covering them with a clean towel dampened with cool tap water. Don't wear contacts until any vision changes have gone away. Don't rub your eyes.

Seek medical care for large blisters or those on the face, hands or genitals. Also seek medical help if you have worsening pain, headache, confusion, nausea, fever, chills, eye pain or vision changes, or signs of infection, such as blisters with swelling, pus or streaks.

NATURE-FRIENDLY SUNSCREEN

Many chemicals found in sunscreens are harmful to coral reef ecosystems. Not only can the chemicals bleach or deform corals, they can impair the growth of green algae, an essential part of the food web. And it's not just the ocean — sunscreen chemicals can negatively affect organisms in all bodies of water. Even if you're nowhere near the ocean, chances are there will be living organisms in the lake you jump into or the stream you stop by.

While some states have started to ban the sale of these sunscreens, they're still making their way to store shelves — sometimes with deceiving labels. So, finding the "good stuff" can be a little tricky. Here are some tips to help:

+ Check the ingredients label. Look for zinc oxide and titanium dioxide (and nothing else).
+ Avoid oxybenzone, octocrylene, avobenzone, benzophenone-1, benzophenone-8, OD-PABA, 4-methylbenzylidene camphor, 3-benzylidene camphor, homosalate, octinoxate, octisalate and nanoparticles.
+ Slather, don't spray. Many spray sunscreens contain harmful nanoparticles.
+ Watch out for green-washing. Some companies will take out just one harmful chemical and slap on a reef-friendly sticker. Go the extra mile and check the ingredients.

BURNS CAUSED BY LIGHTNING

Though it's a rare occurrence to be struck by lightning, it can happen. A lightning strike sends an electrical shock through the body, which can cause burns, heart-rhythm problems, respiratory failure, numbness and tingling, seizures, unconsciousness or cardiac arrest.

A burn caused by lightning may appear minor, but the damage can extend deep into the tissues beneath the skin. Electrical shocks can sometimes result in heart-rhythm disturbance, cardiac arrest or other internal damage from the current passing through the body. Sometimes, the jolt associated with the electrical shock can cause the person to be thrown or to fall, resulting in fractures or other injuries. Observe whether the person is in pain, confused or experiencing changes in their breathing, heartbeat or consciousness. If they are, seek medical attention immediately.

Giving first aid to a person who's been struck by lightning while waiting for professional medical attention can save their life. It's safe to touch a person who's been struck by lightning — the person *does not* carry an electrical charge.

TREATMENT » LIGHTNING STRIKE

1. **Call for help.** Call 911 if you're within cell range or activate the SOS button on an emergency device. Give directions to your location and information about the person. It's safe to use a cellphone or satellite phone during a storm.

PAGE 70

2. **Assess the situation.** Safety is a priority. Be aware of the continued lightning danger to both the person who has been struck and yourself. If located in a high-risk area (for example, near an isolated tree or in an open field), you could be in danger. If necessary, move to a safer location.

   » It's unusual for a person who's survived a lightning strike to have any major broken bones that would cause paralysis or major bleeding complications, unless the person suffered a fall or was thrown a long distance. Therefore, it might be safe to move the person to reduce the risk of further exposure to lightning. Don't move people who are bleeding or appear to have broken bones.

3. **Respond.** Lightning can cause a heart attack. Check to see if the person is breathing and has a heartbeat. The best places to check for a pulse are the carotid artery in the neck or the femoral artery in the groin (see page 175).

   » If the person is breathing normally, look for other possible injuries. Lightning can cause burns, shock, and sometimes blunt trauma. Treat each of these injuries with basic first aid until help arrives.

4. **Resuscitate.** If the person isn't breathing, immediately begin mouth-to-mouth rescue breaths. If they don't have a pulse, start chest compressions as well (CPR). Continue resuscitation efforts until help arrives.

LIGHTNING SAFETY OUTDOORS

Lightning is common in the summer months; however, it can strike any time of the year. The best way to protect yourself from a lightning strike is to avoid the threat. If you hear thunder, you're close enough to be struck by lightning. Remember: There is *no place* outside that's safe during a thunderstorm!

If you absolutely cannot get to safety, you can lessen the threat of being struck with the following tips:

+ Keep moving towards safe shelter. If you're caught out in the open, don't stop.
+ Stay away from isolated trees or other tall objects. If you're in a forest, stay near a lower group of trees.
+ Avoid open fields, hills, boulder fields, rocky outcrops, and ridge tops.
+ Don't lie flat on the ground.
+ Stay away from water, wet items, such as ropes, and metal objects, such as fences and poles.
+ If you're in a group, spread out to prevent the current from traveling between group members.
+ If you're camping in an open area, set up camp in a valley, ravine or other low area. Remember, a tent offers *no* protection from lighting.

5

BLEEDING

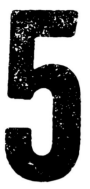

hen an injury results in bleeding, you want to take steps to stop the loss of blood. Most injuries don't cause life-threatening bleeding, but if substantial amounts of blood are lost, shock, unconsciousness and death can result. Appropriate care must be taken to stop the bleeding and also to avoid infection and other complications.

BLEEDING FROM AN OPEN WOUND

Bleeding can range from very minor, such as a needle prick, to major, as with a deep gash in which an artery is severed. All wounds require appropriate care and treatment. Inadequate wound care can result in serious infection. An important precaution against infection is to make sure your tetanus immunization is always up to date.

TYPES OF BLEEDING

When you're assisting someone who's bleeding, it's often helpful to determine the type of bleeding that's occurring because treatment varies. The three main classifications are:

Capillary bleeding

Capillaries are the smallest blood vessels in the body and they're the most numerous. When a minor cut or skin scrape opens one or more capillaries, the bleeding is usually slow and small in volume. The body's normal clotting action generally stops the bleeding in a matter of minutes.

Venous bleeding

Deeper cuts often open veins, releasing blood that's on its way back to the heart. Having delivered its load of oxygen to the body's cells, the blood is dark red. It flows steadily but relatively slowly. Placing firm, direct pressure on the wound will usually stop the blood flow.

Arterial bleeding

The least common but most serious type of bleeding is caused by injury to an artery. The blood that's released is bright red and often spurts with each contraction of the heart. If a major artery is severed and not treated promptly, it's possible to bleed to death within a few minutes. In most cases, however, direct, firm pressure on the wound will stop arterial bleeding.

SEVERE BLEEDING

If your cut is serious — the bleeding doesn't stop on its own in a few minutes or the cut is large or deep — seek emergency medical care. First, stop the bleeding by applying pressure directly to the injury, using a sterile gauze pad or a clean cloth. Maintain pressure until the bleeding stops.

TREATMENT » SEVERE BLEEDING

1. **Lay the bleeding person down.** If possible, elevate the legs.
2. **Don't remove any objects impaled in the person.** Your main concern is to stop the bleeding.
3. **Apply firm pressure directly on the wound.** Use a sterile bandage, clean gauze or even a piece of clothing. If nothing else is available, use your hand. Continuous, firm, direct pressure is your best tool to stop the bleeding.
4. **Maintain pressure until the bleeding stops.** Hold continuous pressure for at least 20 minutes without looking to see if the bleeding has stopped. Maintain pressure afterward, if possible, by binding the wound tightly with a bandage or a piece of clean clothing and adhesive tape. Don't wrap tape all the way around an arm or leg, since this can stop blood flow to it.
5. **Don't remove the gauze or bandage.** If the bleeding continues and seeps through the

PAGE 76

gauze or other material that you're holding on the wound, don't remove it. Instead, add more absorbent material on top of it and maintain firm, direct pressure.

6. **Squeeze the main artery if necessary.** If bleeding of a limb doesn't stop with direct pressure, you may need to make a tourniquet and apply it to the affected limb above the wound (see page 78).

   » Application of a tourniquet should be a last resort when other attempts to stop bleeding have failed.

7. **Immobilize the injured area using a splint, if possible, once the bleeding has stopped**. For bleeding that's difficult to stop, leave the bandages in place and seek immediate emergency care.

PUNCTURE WOUNDS

It's best not to run into a cactus or a porcupine. And don't stomp that tent stake into the ground with your foam sandals. A puncture wound doesn't usually cause much bleeding — a little blood flows and the wound seems to close almost instantly. This doesn't mean that treatment is unnecessary.

Puncture wounds are dangerous because of the risk of infection. The object that caused the wound, especially if it's been exposed to soil, may carry spores of tetanus or other bacteria. These can result in serious infections. A puncture wound through a shoe is particularly prone to serious bacterial infection.

Stopping severe bleeding

If your cut is serious — the bleeding doesn't stop on its own in a few minutes or the cut is large or deep — seek emergency medical care.

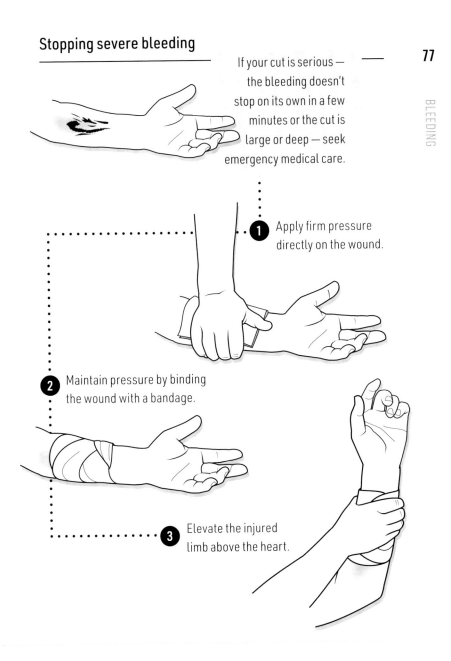

1 Apply firm pressure directly on the wound.

2 Maintain pressure by binding the wound with a bandage.

3 Elevate the injured limb above the heart.

APPLYING A TOURNIQUET

1. Wrap a piece of cloth around the tissue immediately above — but not touching — the wound. The cloth must be long enough to wrap the area twice with enough material left for a knot.

2. Tie a half-knot first, then place a stick or similar object on top of the knot and tie the second half-knot.

3. Twist the stick or object to tighten the tourniquet. Tighten only as much as is required to stop the flow of blood.

4. Note the time you applied the tourniquet.

5. Once the bleeding has stopped, tie the stick in place with the cloth.

6. Try to get to a medical center within two hours of tourniquet application.

BLEEDING

1. **Wash your hands.** This helps prevent infection.
2. **Stop the bleeding.** Apply gentle pressure with a clean bandage or cloth.
3. **Clean the wound.** Rinse the wound with clear water for 5 to 10 minutes. If dirt or debris remains in the wound, use a clean cloth to gently scrub it off.
4. **Apply an ointment.** Apply a thin layer of an antibiotic cream or ointment. For the first two days, rewash the area and reapply the antibiotic when you change the dressing. If a rash appears, stop using the product and seek medical care. Some people develop an allergic reaction to antibiotic cream or ointment. Instead, use petroleum jelly.
5. **Cover the wound.** Bandages help keep the wound clean.
6. **Change the dressing.** Do this daily or whenever the bandage becomes wet or dirty.
7. **Watch for signs of infection.** Seek medical care if the wound isn't healing or you experience increasing pain, pus, swelling or a fever.

Seek medical care if there are signs of infection, such as:
+ Fever.
+ Redness or discoloration, swelling, warmth or increasing pain around the wound.

PAGE 80

+ A bad smell coming from the wound.
+ Pus coming out of the wound.
+ Red streaks around the wound or going up the arm or leg.

Also seek medical care if the wound:
+ Keeps bleeding after a few minutes of direct pressure.
+ Is due to an animal or human bite.
+ Is deep and dirty.
+ Is caused by a metal object.
+ Is deep or dirty and to the head, neck, scrotum, chest or abdomen.
+ Is over a joint and could be deep.

If you haven't had a tetanus shot in the past five years and the wound is deep or dirty, you may need a booster shot. This should happen within 48 hours of the injury.

If the wound was caused by an animal, see page 57 for appropriate treatment.

ABDOMINAL WOUNDS

Any wound that penetrates the abdominal wall is a potentially serious injury because it can injure internal organs. If you or someone with you sustains an abdominal wound, seek emergency medical care.

1. **Lay the bleeding person down.** Before moving someone with an abdominal wound, position the person on their back.
2. **Stop the bleeding.** If no internal organs protrude through the wound, use a gauze pad or sterile cloth and exert pressure on the injury to stop the bleeding. When the blood flow has stopped, tape the bandage in place. If organs are protruding, don't try to replace them in the abdominal cavity.
3. **Bandage the wound.** Cover the injury with a clean dressing.

BLEEDING FROM BODY OPENINGS

Bleeding from body openings can result from an internal injury. Internal bleeding also may accompany seemingly superficial injuries. For example, a blow to the head from a falling rock can produce minor external bleeding, but there may also be internal bleeding. Sometimes an internal injury may show no external signs.

VOMITING BLOOD

Vomiting of blood can occur as the result of injury to the throat, esophagus, stomach or small intestine.

Call 911 if you're within cell range or activate the SOS button on an emergency device. While waiting for help to arrive:

1. **Have the person lie down with their legs elevated, if possible.** Turn the person on their side if the person is vomiting or having trouble breathing to prevent choking.
2. **Don't let the person eat or drink anything.**

COUGHING UP BLOOD

When a person coughs up blood, the source of the blood is usually the lungs or windpipe. The blood that appears may be frothy and bright red. Possible causes include an injury to the chest or lungs.

Seek emergency help if the person coughs up large amounts of blood. While waiting for help to arrive:

1. **Elevate the head.** The person's head should be elevated slightly and supported by padding.
2. **Loosen clothing.** Look for clothing that's tight around the throat, chest or waist.

NOSEBLEEDS

A nosebleed usually involves bleeding from one nostril. It may result from trauma, dry air, allergies or no apparent reason. Most nosebleeds come from the septum, the cartilage that separates the nostrils and is lined with fragile blood vessels. This form of nosebleed isn't serious and is usually easy to stop. In some people, nosebleeds may begin farther back in the nose. These nosebleeds, which are less common, are often harder to stop.

Most often, nosebleeds are only annoying and not a medical problem. But they can be both. Seek medical care if:

+ A nosebleed involves more blood than expected, as can happen in people who take blood-thinning medication.
+ A nosebleed lasts longer than 30 minutes.
+ You feel faint or lightheaded.
+ The nosebleed follows a fall or an accident.

TREATMENT » NOSEBLEEDS

1. **Sit up and lean forward.** Lean forward so blood doesn't go down your throat. This could cause you to choke or have an upset stomach. Don't tilt your head up.
2. **Gently blow your nose.** This will clear blood clots.
3. **Pinch your nose.** Use the thumb and a finger to pinch both nostrils shut just below the bridge of the nose. Breathe through your mouth. Keep pinching for 10 to 15 minutes. Pinching puts pressure on the blood vessels and helps stop the blood

PAGE 84

flow. If the bleeding doesn't stop, pinch the nose again for up to 15 minutes. Seek medical care if the bleeding doesn't stop after the second try.

4. **Prevent another nosebleed.** Don't pick or blow your nose. And don't drop your head below the level of your heart or lift anything heavy for several hours after the nosebleed. Gently put a saline gel, petroleum jelly or an antibiotic ointment on the inside of the nose. Put most of the salve on the middle part of the nose (septum). An ice pack across the bridge of the nose also may help.

5. **If you have another nosebleed, try these steps again.** Seek medical help if the bleeding doesn't stop.

NOSEBLEED » SELF-CARE
Sit up and lean forward. Use the thumb and a finger to pinch both nostrils shut. Breathe through the mouth. Keep pinching for 10 to 15 minutes.

INTERNAL BLEEDING

In the event of a traumatic injury, internal bleeding may not be immediately apparent. Consider it a possibility if you observe any of the following signs or symptoms:

+ Bleeding from the ears, nose, rectum or vagina
+ Vomiting or coughing up blood
+ Bruising on the neck, chest or abdomen
+ Wounds that have penetrated the skull, chest or abdomen
+ Abdominal tenderness, possibly accompanied by rigid or tense abdominal muscles
+ Fractures

Internal bleeding may produce shock. See page 176 for signs of shock and treatment steps. If you suspect internal bleeding, get immediate emergency help.

TREATMENT » INTERNAL BLEEDING

Call 911 if you're within cell range or activate the SOS button on an emergency device. While waiting for help:

1. **Try to keep the person still.** Also loosen the person's clothing.
2. **In case of internal bleeding within an arm or leg, apply direct pressure to the area to stop the bleeding.** You may need to manually compress a major artery between the heart and the fracture or bruise (see page 175).

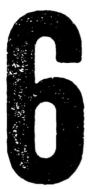

6

POISONING

POISON CENTER » 1-800-222-1222

fraid of getting poisoned in the wilderness? Don't eat plants, berries or mushrooms that you can't identify. Don't drink untreated water from a stream that's right next to a horse trail, and maybe throw out those burger patties that have been sitting in the now-iceless cooler for days. To avoid carbon monoxide poisoning, only use a camp stove in a well-ventilated area, never inside a tent.

Any substance swallowed, inhaled, or absorbed by the body that interferes with its normal function is, by definition, a poison. If you suspect someone has been poisoned, look for evidence, like a person holding a half-eaten mushroom that you can't identify, the spoiled smell of unrefrigerated food, or white gas that's been spilled onto the food stash.

+ Burning sensation or redness around the mouth and lips
+ Breath that smells like chemicals
+ Difficulty breathing
+ Nausea, with or without vomiting
+ Drowsiness
+ Confusion
+ Abdominal or chest pain
+ Uncontrollable restlessness, agitation or having seizures

POISON CENTER » 1-800-222-1222

Call this toll-free number to reach a poison center in the U.S. It's free, confidential and available 24 hours a day.

When you call a poison center, have the following information ready, if possible:

+ The poisoned person's condition, age and weight
+ The ingredients listed on the product container
+ The approximate time the poisoning took place

A poison center isn't a hospital or treatment center. It's a call center staffed by experts on poisoning. The information they can offer may be crucial for delivering fast, appropriate treatment in a poisoning emergency.

The treatment response will depend on the type of poisoning, but in general, the following steps can be taken.

TREATMENT » POISONING

1. **Find fresh air.** If the person has been exposed to poisonous fumes, such as carbon monoxide (while cooking inside a tent, for example), get them into fresh air immediately.

2. **Monitor vital signs.** Be alert for changes in the person who's been poisoned. If breathing stops, begin CPR.

3. **Watch for symptoms of shock.** (See page 176 for signs of shock and treatment steps.)

4. **If the poison has spilled on the person's skin or eyes, flush with plenty of water.** You may need to hold the person's eyelids open while flushing the eyes.

5. **Don't administer ipecac syrup to induce vomiting.** And don't allow the person to eat or drink anything unless instructed to do so.

6. **Call a poison center.** If you happen to be within cell range, call this toll-free number to reach a poison center in the U.S.: 1-800-222-1222.

7. **Seek help.** Call 911 if you're within cell range or activate the SOS button on an emergency device.

CARBON MONOXIDE POISONING

If it's cold or raining outside, don't give in to the temptation to use a camp stove inside an unventilated area, like a tent. Carbon monoxide is colorless and odorless and causes death without warning. Dangerous levels of carbon monoxide can accumulate in as little as 30 minutes inside a tent, and the effects of carbon monoxide become more pronounced at higher altitudes. Always use a camp stove or wood-burning stove outside.

SIGNS AND SYMPTOMS » CARBON MONOXIDE POISONING

+ Headache
+ Weakness
+ Dizziness
+ Nausea or vomiting
+ Shortness of breath
+ Confusion
+ Drowsiness
+ Seizures
+ Loss of consciousness

TREATMENT » CARBON MONOXIDE POISONING

1. **Turn off the carbon monoxide source,** if you can safely do so.
2. **If the person is awake,** get them into fresh air.

3. **If the person is breathing but unresponsive,** try to move them away from the carbon monoxide area into fresh air or ventilate the area by opening tent or cabin doors and windows.
4. **If the person isn't breathing,** begin CPR.

FOODBORNE ILLNESSES

All foods naturally contain small amounts of bacteria. Poor refrigeration, handling or storage can result in bacteria multiplying in large enough numbers to cause illness. That's why it's a good idea to pack nonperishable foods when adventuring outdoors. Ice melts and ice packs thaw, but bacteria stick around.

Signs and symptoms of food poisoning vary depending on the sources of contamination but generally occur within hours after eating the culprit. Whether you become ill after eating contaminated food depends on the amount of exposure, your age and your health. Foodborne illnesses usually improve on their own within 48 hours, but it's important to stay hydrated.

SIGNS AND SYMPTOMS » FOODBORNE ILLNESS

+ Cramping and pain in the abdomen
+ Vomiting
+ Diarrhea (can be bloody)
+ Nausea
+ Fever

1. **Rest.** Avoid any strenuous activities.
2. **Drink plenty of fluids.** Electrolyte drinks help with hydration.
3. **Don't use over-the-counter antidiarrheal medicines.** They can slow the elimination of the bacteria and toxins from your system. Bloody diarrhea typically requires medical treatment.

PREVENT FOOD POISONING

To prevent foodborne illness, practice proper hygiene and safe food-handling:

+ Wash your hands with soap and water or a sanitizing wipe or gel. Do this after going to the bathroom, before eating and before and after handling food.
+ Thaw meats and frozen foods in a cooler stocked with plenty of ice or frozen ice packs and not out in the open.
+ Don't pack dented metal cans or jars with bulging lids.
+ Rinse produce thoroughly with purified water, or peel off the skin or outer leaves (you can do this before you leave home).
+ Wash knives and cutting surfaces with soap and water, especially after handling raw meat and before preparing other foods that will be eaten raw.
+ Cook fish until it flakes easily with a fork.
+ Cook eggs until the yolks are firm.

+ Always check the expiration date on food before you pack it.

+ Don't leave high-risk foods, such as mayonnaise-based egg or potato salads or cream-based sauces, outside a cooler for more than two hours.

+ Discard moldy food.

+ When in doubt, throw it out. If you aren't sure if food has been prepared, served or stored safely, discard it. Even if it looks and smells fine, it may not be safe to eat.

+ Wash dishes thoroughly after each use. Don't wash dishes directly in a body of water like a lake or stream. Instead, dig a hole and use biodegradable soap to wash dishes over the hole. Fill in the hole when done.

+ When you return home, clean and sanitize your cooler. Make a cleaning solution of 1 tablespoon of baking soda and 1 quart of water.

WATERBORNE ILLNESSES

As tempting as it might be to drink straight from glacial melt high in the mountains, it's best to treat all water before consumption to avoid an illness that could ruin your adventure.

Waterborne illnesses are caused by ingesting water contaminated by microscopic viruses or bacteria or water that comes in contact with feces. Bacteria and parasites in contaminated water can cause a variety of waterborne illnesses, some of which might not manifest symptoms until days after infection.

+ Diarrhea (most common symptom)
+ Vomiting
+ Nausea
+ Stomach cramps
+ Bloating
+ Fever
+ Fatigue

HOW TO PURIFY WATER

It's very important that you plan for your water needs, as potable water may not always be available, especially in backcountry and wilderness areas. "Potable water" is clean water that's safe to drink, wash your hands with and use for preparing food. Before you head out, learn about any water quality alerts, such as harmful algal bacteria, that would affect water use.

Never drink water from a natural source that you haven't purified, even if the water looks clean. Water in a stream, river or lake may look clean, but it may be filled with bacteria, viruses and parasites that can cause disease. It's essential that you purify natural water. Purifying water involves filtering it to remove large particles and boiling it or treating it with chemicals to kill organisms.

If you plan to use natural water during your adventure, follow these steps to collect and purify the water.

Step 1: Collect water from your source

The first step is to safely collect the water you'll use. To collect water from a natural source:

1. Start with a clean container.
2. Wash your hands with soap and water or use hand sanitizer before collecting water so you don't contaminate it.
3. Chose a collection spot that's:
   » At a higher elevation or near the water's source.
   » Away from established campsites.
   » Away from animal grazing areas.
4. Collect water from areas of moving water in rivers and streams, or from the top few inches of a lake. Stagnant (standing or non-moving) water should be avoided.
5. Dip your bottle just under the surface to fill it.

Step 2: Filter the water

The next step in the water purification process is filtration. Filtration by itself doesn't purify water. It must be followed by boiling or disinfection to purify it for drinking.

+ Most water filters contain a screen with many tiny holes in it. These filters can remove protozoa and some bacteria, but they can't filter out viruses.

+ Filters also remove bigger contaminants like leaves, silt, dirt and sand. If the water is cloudy or has floating material in it, filter it even if you plan to boil or disinfect it.

+ Be sure to use and care for your filter according to the manufacturer's instructions. Filters don't work as well if they aren't taken care of over time.

Step 3: Disinfect the water

The final step of purification is disinfecting the water, which can be done by either boiling it or treating it with a disinfectant. This is the most important step, as these methods will kill any remaining organisms in the water, especially those that could make you sick.

Boiling

Boiling is the best way to kill disease-causing organisms. The high temperature and time spent boiling are very important to effectively kill organisms in the water. Boiling will also effectively treat water if it's still cloudy or murky.

To prepare your water for drinking, put the water in a container over a heat source, such as a campfire or propane stove, and bring it to a rolling boil following these guidelines:

+ If you're at an elevation below 6,500 feet, bring the water to a rolling boil for 1 minute.
+ If you're at an elevation above 6,500 feet, bring the water to a rolling boil for 3 minutes.

WARNING You might want to talk to a medical professional before using disinfection products. Some tablets or drops, especially iodine, may not be safe for pregnant women, people with thyroid issues or iodine hypersensitivities, or for use over long periods of time.

Disinfection

Disinfection happens when a chemical or UV light is added to water to kill bacteria, viruses and other potentially harmful organisms. Many factors can impact the effectiveness of these methods, including water temperature, pH and cloudiness. With disinfectants, it's important to allow the chemical or UV light enough time to treat the water and kill any organisms before drinking — this is called contact time.

Chemical disinfection involves adding one or more chemicals effective at killing waterborne organisms to your filtered water.

+ Chemical tablets or liquid drops are the most common ways to disinfect natural water. Iodine or chlorine dioxide are the most frequently used disinfection agents. Products approved by the National Sanitation Foundation (NSF) are recommended.

+ Follow the manufacturer's instructions for disinfecting the water. Contact time to disinfect the water varies by product and can range from 30 minutes to several hours. If the water is cloudy or has floating debris, it will be more effective to pre-filter the water before disinfecting.

POISONOUS PLANTS

Wild mushrooms, berries and other plants can be delicious treats outdoors. Misidentifying them, however, can be bad news for your digestive system — or even deadly.

Certain plants are poisonous only when ingested. Be aware of common poisonous plants in the areas where you adventure, and educate the people you're with, especially children. In general, unless you know for certain they're safe, don't eat berries of any color, especially those on plants with bitter smells, spines or milky sap. A good rule of thumb: When in doubt, don't eat it.

If you think someone has ingested a poisonous plant, seek emergency medical help. Get a sample of the plant or take a photo of the leaves or berries, if there are any. If you're within cell range, call the nearest poison center for steps you can take while you wait for help (1-800-222-1222).

SIGNS AND SYMPTOMS » INGESTING POISONOUS PLANTS

+ Burning pain in the mouth and throat
+ Swelling in the throat that may lead to difficulty breathing
+ Vomiting
+ Abdominal pain or diarrhea
+ Hallucinations
+ Seizures
+ Unconsciousness

DON'T TOUCH THESE PLANTS

Certain plants have surface oils that irritate skin. To avoid brushing up against any of these plants, stick to the trail and avoid bushwhacking. Familiarize yourself with the characteristics of common poisonous plants so you're quick to identify them. The saying "Leaves of three, let it be!" is a helpful reminder.

Respiratory problems can also arise if you burn certain kinds of poisonous plants. So, before you add that branch to the campfire, take a closer look.

TREATMENT » SKIN CONTACT

1. **Wash up.** Clean your skin right away with soap and water. Scrub under your nails with a brush.
2. **Don't scratch.** Scratching can cause infection and can also transfer the oils elsewhere on the body.
3. **Leave blisters alone.** If blisters open, don't remove the overlying skin.
4. **Relieve the itch.** Apply calamine lotion, hydrocortisone cream or wet compresses.
5. **Take an oral antihistamine.** Follow directions on the package, and be aware that some antihistamines can make you drowsy.

WARNING The plants and fruits shown in this chapter are meant to alert you to potentially dangerous species you may encounter during your adventures. This book is not an official field guide and shouldn't be used as such.

The best way to keep from getting sick from poisonous plants and fruits is not to eat them, even if you believe you've identified a type that's safe to consume.

DON'T EAT THESE PLANTS

BITTER NIGHTSHADE

Clusters of green berries that ripen to bright red. Flowers appear in clusters and hang downward; bright purple petals with protruding yellow stamens in center.

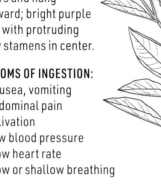

SYMPTOMS OF INGESTION:
+ Nausea, vomiting
+ Abdominal pain
+ Salivation
+ Low blood pressure
+ Slow heart rate
+ Slow or shallow breathing

BITTERSWEET

Drooping clusters of orange fruits, approximately pea-sized. Small, greenish flowers at the tips of branches.

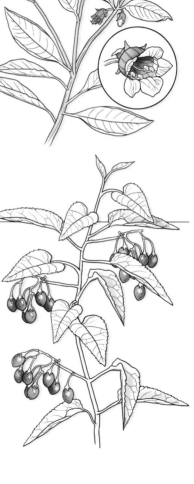

SYMPTOMS OF INGESTION:
+ Vomiting
+ Diarrhea
+ Loss of consciousness
+ Seizures

FOXGLOVE

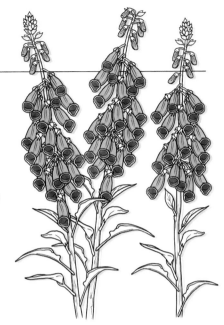

Clusters of bell-shaped flowers, usually bright purple; numerous dark spots on inner surface.

SYMPTOMS OF INGESTION:
+ Nausea, vomiting
+ Irregular and slow pulse
+ Tremors
+ Seeing unusual colors
+ Convulsions
+ Irregular heartbeats

HOLLY

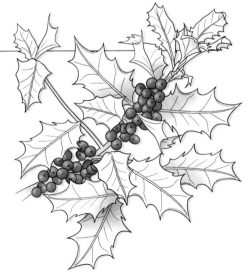

Small berries, bright red or bright yellow. Thick, dark-green leaves with spiny teeth along edges.

SYMPTOMS OF INGESTION:
+ Vomiting
+ Diarrhea
+ Depression

DON'T EAT THESE PLANTS

VIRGINIA CREEPER

Blue-black berries,
usually hidden by five
saw-toothed leaflets.

SYMPTOMS OF INGESTION:
+ Abdominal pain
+ Bloody vomiting
  or diarrhea
+ Sweating
+ Weak pulse
+ Drowsiness
+ Twitching
  of the face

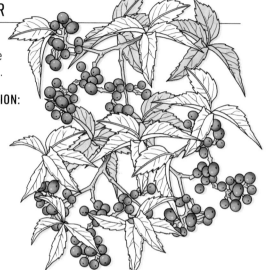

YEW

Evergreen tree with dense
branches with dark-green,
needle-like leaves.
Fruits are bright red,
berry-like structures.

SYMPTOMS OF INGESTION:
+ Dry mouth
+ Vertigo
+ Abdominal pain
+ Difficulty breathing
+ Irregular heart rhythm
+ Low blood pressure
+ Cardiac and respiratory
  failure can occur

DANGEROUS MUSHROOMS

WARNING Poisonous wild mushrooms can be almost impossible to tell apart from those that aren't poisonous, and many cases of poisoning have happened in people who had a lot of experience and were "sure" they had picked the right kind of mushroom. Likewise, folklore isn't a reliable way to avoid poisonous mushrooms.

Some of the deadliest wild mushrooms don't cause obvious symptoms for hours or even days or weeks after they're eaten, and, by the time symptoms appear, it's very possible that liver or kidney damage has already occurred.

The mushrooms shown in this chapter are meant to highlight some of the most dangerous ones that you may encounter during your adventures. As stated previously, this book is not an official field guide on identifying poisonous plants.

The best way to keep from getting sick from wild mushrooms is not to eat them, even if you believe you've identified a type that's safe to consume.

DANGEROUS MUSHROOMS

AUTUMN SKULLCAP

Brownish cap with yellowish gills; ring on brown stalk.

TOXICITY: Deadly

SYMPTOMS:
+ Severe abdominal pain
+ Persistent vomiting
+ Diarrhea
+ Extreme thirst
+ Apparent recovery after a few hours lasting up to five days, followed by signs and symptoms of liver or kidney dysfunction

DEADLY CORT

Deep orange-brown cap and stalk with remnants of yellow veil.

TOXICITY: Deadly

SYMPTOMS: Appear a minimum of three days up to three weeks after ingestion
+ Thirst
+ Frequent urination
+ Loss of appetite
+ Feeling cold
+ Signs and symptoms of kidney failure

NOTE: Particularly dangerous because of the characteristic long delay in the occurrence of symptoms.

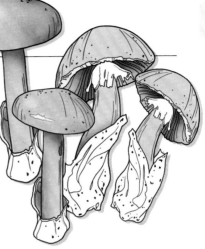

DEATH CAP

Smooth, greenish cap with skirt-like ring at top of stalk and sac-like cup at base.

TOXICITY: Deadly

SYMPTOMS:
Appear 6-12 hours after ingestion
+ Severe abdominal pain
+ Persistent vomiting
+ Diarrhea
+ Extreme thirst
+ Apparent recovery after a few hours lasting up to five days, followed by indications of liver or kidney dysfunction

DESTROYING ANGEL

White with flaring to ragged ring on stalk; large, sac-like cup at base.

TOXICITY: Deadly

SYMPTOMS: Appear 6-12 hours after ingestion
+ Severe abdominal pain
+ Persistent vomiting
+ Diarrhea
+ Extreme thirst
+ Apparent recovery after a few hours lasting up to five days, followed by indications of liver or kidney dysfunction

DANGEROUS MUSHROOMS

FALSE MOREL

Brownish, brain-like or saddle-shaped cap on short, whitish stalk.

TOXICITY: Deadly

SYMPTOMS: Appear approximately six hours after ingestion
+ Sudden onset of abdominal discomfort
+ Severe headache
+ Vomiting

NOTE: Often mistaken for the nonpoisonous morel mushroom.

JACK O'LANTERN

Orange to yellowish-orange mushroom with sharp-edged gills descending stalk.

TOXICITY: Poisonous

SYMPTOMS: Appear 1-6 hours after ingestion
+ Nausea
+ Vomiting
+ Diarrhea

NOTE: Often mistaken for the chanterelle mushroom. When gathered fresh and observed in the dark, gills give off an eerie green glow.

SHAGGY-STALKED LEPIOTA

Small white cap with brownish scales, vanishing ring on shaggy-wooly stalk, gills separate from stalk.

TOXICITY: Poisonous

SYMPTOMS:
Appear hours
after ingestion
+ Nausea
+ Vomiting
+ Diarrhea
+ Stomach cramps
+ Profuse sweating

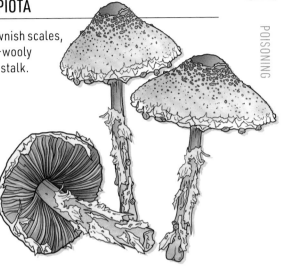

SWEATING MUSHROOM

Small, smooth, dull-white mushroom with gills slightly descending the stalk.

TOXICITY: Poisonous

SYMPTOMS: Appear within 15-20 minutes of ingestion
+ Excessive salivation
+ Sweating
+ Abdominal pains
+ Vomiting
+ Diarrhea
+ Blurred vision
+ Labored breathing

DON'T TOUCH THESE PLANTS

DEADLY NIGHTSHADE

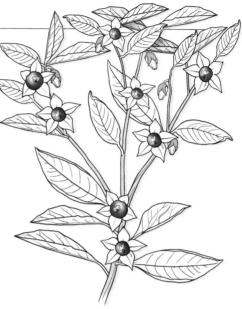

Dark-green leaves with purple bell-shaped, drooping flowers. Berries are glossy black, approximately ½-inch in diameter.

POISONOUS PART: All
*Highest concentration of toxins in berries

SYMPTOMS OF CONTACT:
+ Headache, fever
+ Rapid pulse
+ Difficulty swallowing
+ Hallucinations
+ Convulsions

NOTE: Ingesting the berries is the most harmful, but toxins also can be absorbed through the skin or cause severe dermatitis.

DAPHNE

Pink to purple flowers that
are very fragrant with
bright-red berries.

POISONOUS PART: All
*Highest concentration of
  toxins in berries, twigs and sap

SYMPTOMS OF CONTACT:
+ Skin irritation
+ Swelling of lips and tongue
+ Thirst
+ Weakness

NOTE: May be fatal if eaten.

GIANT HOGWEED

Green stems with dark-red to purple
blemishes and coarse white hairs.
Flat-topped white flowers.

POISONOUS PART: Sap (clear, watery)
found in all parts of the plant

SYMPTOMS OF CONTACT:
+ Painful lesions, including
  severe blisters and burns
+ Inflammatory skin reaction
  induced by sunlight
  (phototoxic dermatitis)
+ Symptoms can persist
  for weeks to months

DON'T TOUCH THESE PLANTS

JERUSALEM CHERRY

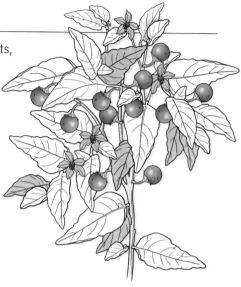

Red, yellow or orange fruits, about the size of a cherry.

POISONOUS PART: All
*Fruit is highly toxic when ingested

SYMPTOMS OF CONTACT:
+ Dermatitis if handled
+ Nausea, vomiting
+ Abdominal pain
+ Salivation
+ Seizures

OLEANDER

Long, narrow, dark-green leaves with five-petaled flowers in a variety of colors.

POISONOUS PART: All

SYMPTOMS OF CONTACT:
+ Nausea, vomiting
+ Irregular heartbeat
+ Dizziness
+ Drowsiness

POISON HEMLOCK

Leaves resemble parsley. Purple blotches on smooth stem; small white flowers in clusters.

POISONOUS PART: All

SYMPTOMS OF CONTACT:
+ Redness or discoloration
+ Inflammation
+ Itching
+ Blistering

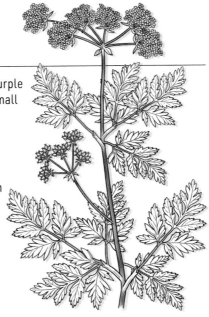

POISON IVY

Leaflets are always in groups of three; middle leaflet is longer than outer two.

POISONOUS PART: All
*Highest concentration of toxins in leaves and bark

SYMPTOMS OF CONTACT:
+ Redness or discoloration
+ Inflammation
+ Itching
+ Blistering

NOTE: Inhaling smoke from burning poison ivy can cause severe respiratory problems.

DON'T TOUCH THESE PLANTS

POISON OAK

Similar to poison ivy, but distinguished by its lobed leaves.

POISONOUS PART: All
*Highest concentration of toxins in leaves and bark

SYMPTOMS OF CONTACT:
+ Redness or discoloration
+ Inflammation
+ Itching
+ Blistering

NOTE: Inhaling smoke from burning poison oak can cause severe respiratory problems.

POISON SUMAC

Smooth, oval leaves; distinctive reddish stems.

POISONOUS PART: All
*Much more allergenic than poison ivy or poison oak

SYMPTOMS OF CONTACT:
+ Redness or discoloration
+ Inflammation
+ Itching
+ Blistering

NOTE: Inhaling smoke from burning poison sumac can cause severe respiratory problems.

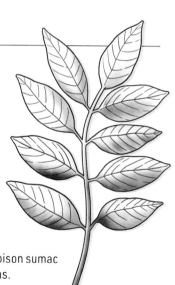

POKEWEED

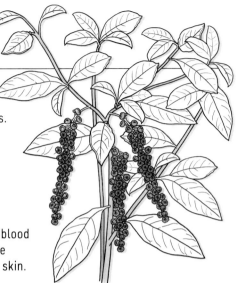

Drooping clusters
of dark blue-black
berries with purple stems.

POISONOUS PART: All

SYMPTOMS OF CONTACT:
+ Dehydration
+ Vomiting

NOTE: May cause serious blood
abnormalities if toxins are
absorbed through cuts in skin.

STINGING NETTLE

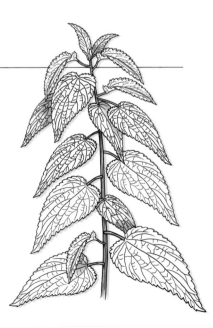

Elongated heart-shaped leaves
with saw-toothed edges;
stems may have stinging hairs.

POISONOUS PART: Leaves, stems

SYMPTOMS OF CONTACT:
+ Intense burning
+ Itching

7

FOREIGN BODIES

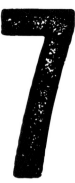

It's hard to ignore that splinter in your palm, that speck of dirt in your eye or that bug in your ear. Children and adults alike can get foreign objects stuck in places they shouldn't. Sometimes it's possible to remove foreign objects from the body without the help of a doctor. Here are some tips to help you do that. If the problem persists, seek medical attention.

IN THE EYES

As if by magic, an eye often protects itself from or gets rid of foreign airborne objects, such as specks of dirt, by reflexively tearing up and blinking. If you have something in your eye and tearing and blinking aren't getting the job done, address the issue promptly to avoid damage from scratches, infection or chemical exposure.

Caution: Don't rub the eye or remove an object that's embedded in it. Seek immediate medical care to remove an embedded object.

1. **Wash up.** Clean your hands with soap and water.
2. **Remove contact lens.** If you wear contact lenses, remove the lens before or while you're irrigating the surface of the eye.
3. **Fill a small cup with water.** Make sure both the cup and water are clean.
4. **Position the cup.** Rest the rim of the cup on the bone at the base of your eye socket.
5. **Pour the water in.** Tilt the cup and keep the eye open.
6. **Take a shower.** If you have access to a shower with clean water, another way to flush a foreign object is to aim a gentle stream of lukewarm water on your forehead over the affected eye while holding your eyelid open.
7. **Monitor symptoms.** Even if you think the object has been removed, flush your eye

To flush your own eye, rest the rim of the cup on the bone at the base of your eye socket.

if it still hurts and looks red. If an object scratches your eye, it may feel as though the object is still in the eye even after it's been removed.

TREATMENT » FLUSHING SOMEONE ELSE'S EYE

1. **Wash up.** Clean your hands with soap and water.
2. **Find good light.** Seat the person in a well-lit area.
3. **Gently examine the eye to find the object.** Pull the lower lid downward and instruct the person to look up, down, left and right, as objects can hide in the recesses of the eye. Then hold the upper eyelid while the person looks down.
4. **Flush it.** If the object is floating in the tear film on the surface of the eye, try flushing it out with clean water by using a medicine dropper filled with water or using a small glass and gently pouring the water into the eye.
5. **Monitor symptoms.**

Similar items can be used in the absence of an eye cup.

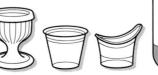

IN THE EARS

Children sometimes stick objects in their ears, such as pebbles, plants or seeds. Adults are guilty of this, too. Remember this rule of thumb: Don't put anything in your ear smaller than your elbow. Occasionally, an uninvited insect will take up residence in your ear. The good news is that you can evict it. Objects in the ears can cause pain or impair hearing, so address the issue promptly.

Caution: If there's bleeding, severe pain, drainage or signs of infection, seek medical care right away.

TREATMENT » REMOVE FROM EAR

1. **Don't probe the ear with any tools, including a cotton swab.** You could push the object farther into the ear and damage the fragile structures of the middle ear.
2. **Use gravity.** Tilt the person's head so the affected side is downward to try to dislodge the object.
3. **Remove the object.** If the object is clearly visible, is pliable and can be easily grasped with tweezers, gently remove it. Be sure to get a firm grip on the object to avoid forcing it farther in.
4. **Use water.** If the person doesn't have a hole in the eardrum or tubes in place, use a rubber-bulb syringe and clean, warm water to wash

the object out of the ear canal. Don't use water
to remove plant material, food or batteries.

5. **Use oil or alcohol.** If the object is an insect, you
can try to float the insect out by pouring a small
amount of alcohol or warm (not hot) olive oil,
baby oil or mineral oil into the ear. Warm the
bottle of oil by rubbing it between your hands.
Don't use alcohol or oil if the person has a hole
in the eardrum or tubes in place.

» Tilt the person's head so the affected ear
is upward.

» To ease the entry of the oil, straighten the
ear canal by grasping the top of the ear and
pulling it slightly back. The insect should
suffocate and may float out in the liquid.

6. **Monitor symptoms.** If these methods fail and
the person continues to experience pain or
reduced hearing, see a doctor as soon as possible.

IN THE NOSE

The nose is a favorite place for children and adult jokesters
to insert objects such as sticks, rocks or food. Sometimes the
objects get stuck.

Caution: If attempts to remove the object are unsuccessful,
seek medical assistance. Delaying removal of the object could
lead to an infection and nasal damage.

119

FOREIGN BODIES

1. **Don't probe the object.** Don't poke at it with a cotton swab, matchstick or other tool, which risks pushing the object farther into the nose.

2. **Don't try to inhale the object forcefully by breathing in.** Instead, breathe through your mouth until the object is removed.

3. **Blow your nose.** Blow short, firm puffs of air while applying gentle pressure to the opposite nostril to close it, forcing the air out the clogged nostril.

4. **Remove the object, if possible.** If the object is clearly visible, is pliable and can be easily grasped with tweezers, gently try to remove it. Be sure to get a firm grip on the object to avoid forcing it farther in.

5. **Perform a "parent's kiss."** Place gentle pressure on the unaffected nostril to close it. Then, firmly seal your mouth around the child's mouth and deliver short puffs of air into the child's mouth. This may dislodge the object.

IN THE WINDPIPE OR LUNGS

When an object is accidentally inhaled, sometimes it lodges in the windpipe or the lungs. Typically, this will cause coughing. If an inhaled object causes choking, use the Heimlich maneuver to dislodge it.

1. **Perform the Heimlich maneuver.** If the person is choking, perform the Heimlich maneuver (see page 128).
2. **Seek emergency care.** If the problem persists, seek medical help as soon as possible.

SWALLOWED

If you swallow a foreign object — like an insect that flies into your mouth while you're mountain biking — it will usually pass through the digestive system without a problem. Sometimes, though, an object can become lodged.

Caution: Get immediate medical care if you, or someone with you, swallows a button battery or magnet, or a sharp or pointed object.

For other objects, seek emergency medical help if the following signs or symptoms appear:

+ Difficulty swallowing
+ Spitting up saliva
+ Chest pain
+ Abdominal pain or vomiting
+ Coughing

IN THE SKIN

It's common for an object to become embedded in your skin. You can often safely remove small foreign objects such as a wood splinter, thorn or small piece of glass just under the skin's surface.

Caution: If the object is close to an eye or deeply embedded, or if it's large or dirty, placing you at risk of infection, seek medical attention.

TREATMENT » PARTIALLY EMBEDDED IN SKIN

1. **Wash up.** Wash your hands and clean the affected area well with soap and water.
2. **Remove the object.** Use tweezers to remove splinters, cactus spines or other foreign objects. If available, use a magnifying glass to see better.

TREATMENT » FULLY EMBEDDED IN SKIN

1. **Wash up.** Wash your hands and clean the area well with soap and water.
2. **Sterilize a clean, sharp needle.** Use rubbing alcohol or wipe it with an antiseptic wipe. If neither are available, use soap and water.
3. **Use the needle to gently break the skin over the object.** Then lift the tip of the object out.

4. **Use tweezers.** Grab the end of the object and remove it, if possible.
5. **Prevent infection.** Wash the area again, pat it dry and apply antibiotic ointment or petroleum jelly.

Seek prompt medical help for a foreign object that is deeply embedded in the skin or muscle. Follow these precautions:

+   **Don't try to remove the object.** Doing so could cause further harm.
+   **Bandage the wound.** First, put a piece of gauze over the object. Then, if it helps, place clean padding around the object before binding the wound securely with a bandage or piece of clean cloth. Take care not to press too hard on the object.

Also seek prompt medical attention if the wound is deep or dirty and it's been more than five years since your last tenanus shot.

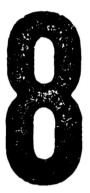

8

CHOKING AND THE HEIMLICH MANEUVER

hoking can happen when a poorly timed joke causes a person to laugh while eating, quickly turning a funny situation into a serious one. Choking occurs in an instant when a piece of food becomes lodged in the windpipe, blocking the flow of air to the lungs. This, in turn, reduces the supply of oxygen-rich blood to the brain and other organs. If the problem isn't corrected quickly, choking can be fatal. A common (though unhelpful) instinct of a choking person is to remove themselves from a social situation, isolating themself from people that can help.

Solid foods, such as meat, are the usual culprits, especially when they're being chewed while the person talks, laughs, eats too fast, walks or runs. Excessive consumption of alcohol can also interfere with swallowing properly, since alcohol is a sedative and dulls the nerves that help you swallow and sense how well your food has been chewed.

A choking person is unable to communicate verbally, so hand gestures become an important way to signal that something is wrong.

+ One or both hands clutching the throat (universal sign for choking)
+ Look of panic, shock or confusion
+ Wheezing, gasping or noisy breathing
+ Inability to speak
+ Inability to cough forcefully
+ Silent cough
+ Skin, lips and nails turning blue or dusky
+ Loss of consciousness

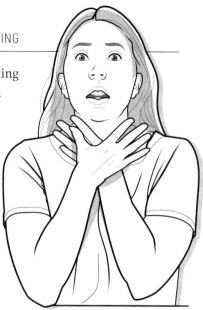

The universal sign for choking.

COUGHING VS. CHOKING

If a morsel of food "goes down the wrong pipe," the coughing reflex will often quickly solve the problem. In fact, a person isn't choking if they're able to cough normally. However, if the cough is silent or more like a gasp, the person is probably choking.

Ask the person if they're choking. If the person indicates yes by nodding their head without speaking, they're choking. If the person can talk, then the airway isn't completely blocked, and oxygen is reaching the lungs. Give them a chance to clear the foreign object by coughing.

HOW TO CLEAR AN OBSTRUCTED AIRWAY

In an unresponsive person, if you can see the food or object causing the blockage and it's at the back of the throat or high in the throat, sweep a finger into the back of the person's throat to clear the airway. Be careful not to push the food or object deeper into the airway, which can happen easily with children. If you can't see the object, don't blindly insert your finger.

In a person who's responsive, clear the obstruction by performing the Heimlich maneuver. The Heimlich should be performed on someone only if there's a complete or near-complete blockage of the airway.

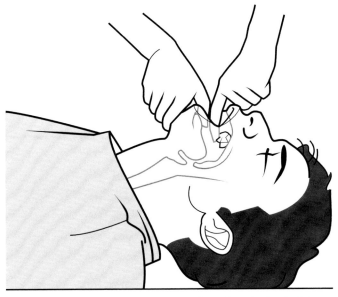

To clear an obstructed airway, sweep a finger into the back of the person's throat.

PERFORMING THE HEIMLICH MANEUVER

You've likely seen the Heimlich maneuver displayed on posters and acted out on television and maybe wondered: Could I do that? Well, if you're in the middle of the ocean or on top of a mountain, faced with an emergency like choking, no doubt you'll rise to the occasion. It's a simple matter of swift action and confidence.

THE HEIMLICH MANEUVER » ON SOMEONE ELSE

1. **Give five back blows.** Stand behind the choking person and bend the person over at the waist to face the ground. Strike five separate times between the person's shoulder blades with the heel of your hand.

2. **Perform the Heimlich maneuver.** If the back blows don't remove the object, get ready to perform the Heimlich maneuver. Stand behind the choking person and wrap your arms around the person's waist. Tilt the person slightly forward.

3. **Make a fist with one hand.** Place the fist slightly above the person's navel.
    » If the person is pregnant or carries excess weight, place your fist at the base of the breastbone, above the belly and right at the joining of the lowest ribs.

4. **Grasp the fist with the other hand.** Press into

the stomach (abdomen) with a quick, upward thrust, as if you were trying to lift the person up.

5. **Give five abdominal thrusts.** These should be done in rapid succession. Check if the blockage has been removed and repeat if needed. Continue until the person either coughs up the object or becomes unresponsive. If they start coughing or cough up the object, let them try to expel it.

6. **Perform CPR.** If the person becomes unresponsive, begin CPR.

The proper hand and arm positioning for performing the Heimlich maneuver on someone else.

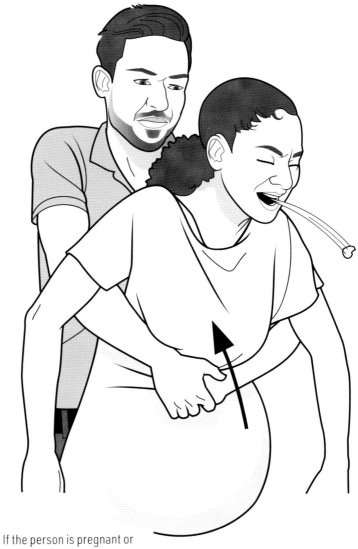

If the person is pregnant or
carries excess weight, place your fist at the base of the
breastbone, above the belly and right at the joining of the lowest ribs.

1. **Make a fist.** Place it slightly above your navel, with the thumb side toward your abdomen.
2. **Grasp and bend.** Grasp your fist with your other hand and bend over a hard or stable surface, such as a picnic table, sturdy camp chair or hiking pole.
3. **Shove your fist inward and upward.** Continue to do so until the object dislodges.

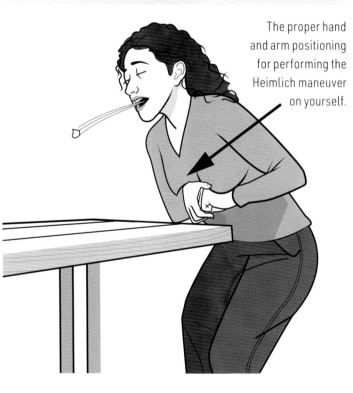

The proper hand and arm positioning for performing the Heimlich maneuver on yourself.

CHOKING AND THE HEIMLICH MANEUVER

For a child younger than age 1, follow these steps.

1. **Sit and hold the infant facedown on your forearm.** Rest your forearm on your thigh. Hold the infant's chin and jaw to support the head. Place the head lower than the trunk.

Gentle but firm thumps on the back can help clear the airway of a choking infant.

MAYO CLINIC FIRST-AID GUIDE FOR OUTDOOR ADVENTURES

2. **Thump the infant gently but firmly five times on the middle of the back.** Use the heel of your hand. Point your fingers up so that you don't hit the back of the infant's head. Gravity and the back thumps should release the blockage.

3. **Turn the infant faceup on your forearm if breathing hasn't started.** Rest your arm on your thigh. Place the infant's head lower than the trunk.

4. **Give five gentle but firm chest compressions with your fingers.** Place two fingers just below the nipple line. Press down about 1½ inches. Let the chest rise between each compression.

5. **Repeat the back thumps and chest compressions if breathing doesn't start.** Call for emergency medical help.

6. **Perform CPR.** Begin infant CPR if the airway is clear but the infant doesn't start breathing.

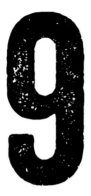

9

CPR

(CARDIOPULMONARY RESUSCITATION)

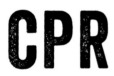

ardiopulmonary resuscitation (CPR) is a real life-saver. It may need to be used in a range of emergencies that can lead to cardiac arrest, such as a heart attack, drowning or lightning strike, or if a person is choking or has been severely burned. Cardiac arrest is when the person doesn't have a pulse and isn't breathing.

CPR can keep oxygenated blood flowing to the brain and other vital organs until an emergency response team arrives.

Performing CPR like a pro means combining two key elements: chest compressions and mouth-to-mouth rescue breathing. Even if you're uncertain whether your knowledge and abilities are sufficient, the bottom line is that it's better to do something than nothing.

Follow this advice from the American Heart Association:

+ **Untrained.** If you're not trained in CPR or if you're worried about giving rescue breaths, then provide hands-only CPR. That means uninterrupted chest compressions at 100 to 120 times a minute until medical help arrives. You don't need to try rescue breathing.

+ **Trained and ready to go.** If you're well-trained and confident in your ability, perform both chest compressions and rescue breathing. Start CPR with 30 chest compressions before giving two rescue breaths.

+ **Trained but rusty.** If you've previously received CPR training but you're not confident in your abilities, just do chest compressions at a rate of 100 to 120 a minute.

BEFORE YOU BEGIN CPR

Before starting CPR, assess the situation:

+ Quickly scan the scene to make sure there aren't imminent hazards to your own personal safety.

+ Check to see if the person is responsive. Tap their shoulder and shout, "Are you OK?"

+ If the person is unresponsive (doesn't answer, moan or move), have someone call 911 if you're within cell range, or use the SOS button on an emergency response device.

+ Check to see if the person is breathing or if their breathing is abnormal (such as gasping).

+ If the person is unresponsive and isn't breathing or has abnormal breathing, the person is likely in cardiac arrest. Immediately begin CPR. It's not necessary to check for a pulse if you're not medically trained.

  » If you've misread the situation and the person does have a pulse, the act of CPR will be painful enough that they'll somehow demonstrate that they're conscious.

  » If the person has a pulse but isn't breathing, performing a head tilt-chin lift can help open the airway (see page 140).

HOW TO PERFORM CPR

When performing CPR, the first and most important step is to do chest compressions.

BEGIN CHEST COMPRESSIONS

Forceful, rhythmic compression of the chest should be started as soon as cardiac arrest is suspected. When you perform chest compressions, you're acting as a pump to push blood and oxygen to the heart and brain.

PERFORM CPR » CHEST COMPRESSIONS

1. **Position the person on their back.** Find a firm surface. Kneel next to the person's shoulders and neck.
2. **Place the heel of one of your hands over the center of the person's chest, between the nipples.** Place your other hand on top of the first hand and interlace your fingers. Keep your elbows straight and position your shoulders directly above your hands.
3. **Push hard and fast (two compressions per second).** Use your upper body weight (not just your arms) as you push down on (compress) the chest between 2 and 2½ inches. Let the chest recoil between compressions.

PAGE 138 ▶

CPR (CARDIOPULMONARY RESUSCITATION)

4. **Continue CPR.** If you're an untrained layperson, continue performing CPR using continuous hard and fast chest compressions — 100 to 120 compressions a minute — until help arrives.

5. **Seek help.** If you're alone and no one else can call 911 or activate the SOS button on an emergency response device, perform about two minutes of compressions before taking a short break to contact emergency personnel.

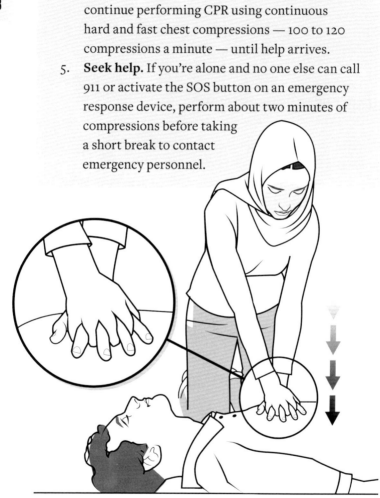

Perform chest compressions by placing one hand over the center of the person's chest and placing your other hand on top of the first hand. Push hard and with a fast tempo.

OPEN THE AIRWAY

If you're trained in CPR and are comfortable giving rescue breaths, then after you've performed 30 chest compressions, open the person's airway. If you don't have CPR training, open the airway after seeking emergency help and before continuing chest compressions.

PERFORM CPR » OPEN THE AIRWAY

1. **Perform the head tilt-chin lift.** Place your palm on the person's forehead and tilt the head back. With the other hand, gently lift the chin forward to open the airway. Don't press deeply into the soft tissue below the chin.

    » **If a spinal injury is suspected, use the modified jaw thrust and not the head tilt-chin lift.** To perform the modified jaw thrust, which protects the neck (cervical spine), use your index and middle fingers to push the lower jaw upward and outward while the thumbs push down on the chin to open the mouth. If another person is available, have that person stabilize the head and neck.

2. **Return to chest compressions or perform rescue breaths.** If you don't have CPR training, resume chest compressions. Otherwise, perform rescue breaths.

If you're trained in CPR:

1. **Make a seal.** With the airway open (using the head-tilt, chin-lift maneuver), pinch the nostrils shut for mouth-to-mouth breathing and cover the person's mouth with yours, making a seal.

2. **Give the first breath, lasting one second, with enough air to make the chest visibly rise.** If it does, give a second rescue breath, also lasting one second.

3. **Repeat if needed.** If the chest doesn't rise, repeat the head tilt-chin lift maneuver or jaw thrust and give another breath.

4. **Check for signs.** If there's no breathing, coughing or movement, resume chest compressions.

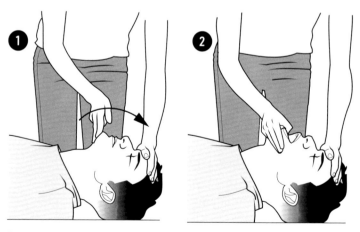

To open the airway, first tilt the head back, and then lift the chin.

The procedure for giving CPR to children (age 1 through puberty) is essentially the same as that for adults, with a few differences.

PERFORM CPR » ON A CHILD

1. **If you're not trained in CPR and don't know how to perform rescue breaths, do compression-only CPR.** If you know how to perform rescue breaths, children may benefit from this step. Cardiac arrest in children is frequently due to a breathing problem.

2. **You may use one or two hands to perform chest compressions, depending on the size of the child.** Push down on the chest at least one-third of its depth (about 2 inches). Push hard and fast — 100 to 120 compressions per minute. Let the chest recoil between compressions.

3. **Open the airway by placing your palm on the child's forehead and gently tilt the head back.** With the other hand, gently lift the chin forward to open the airway.

4. **If you're performing rescue breaths, breathe more gently, but make sure the child's chest rises.** Each breath should take about one second. As with adults, alternate

PAGE 142

between 30 chest compressions and two rescue breaths.

5. **If you're alone** and no one else can call 911 or activate the SOS button on an emergency response device, perform about two minutes of compressions or five cycles of compressions and breaths before leaving the child momentarily to alert emergency personnel.

6. **Continue performing CPR** until the child moves or help arrives.

SPECIFIC EMERGENCIES

Physical exertion can increase the risk of a variety of medical emergencies, so familiarize yourself with your adventure companions' medical histories before heading outdoors. Make sure everyone has their medications and that they understand the assumed risk.

HEART ATTACK

Some heart attacks strike suddenly, but many people have warning signs hours or days in advance. A heart attack generally causes chest pain for more than 15 minutes. If you think you or someone in your group is having a heart attack, follow these steps:

1. **Seek emergency help**. Call 911 if you're within cell range or activate the SOS button on an emergency device.

2. **Chew and swallow aspirin.** Do this while waiting for emergency help to arrive. Aspirin keeps your blood from clotting, and when taken during a heart attack could reduce heart damage. It's important to chew the tablet — one 324 mg tablet or four 81 mg tablets — no matter how bad it tastes.

3. **Take nitroglycerin, if prescribed.** If you think you're having a heart attack and your doctor has previously prescribed nitroglycerin for you, take it as directed while waiting for emergency help.

4. **Report medical history.** Inform your travel companions about any heart or medical conditions you have so they can relay this information to the dispatch operator.

5. **Don't drive.** If you're near your vehicle, don't drive yourself to seek emergency medical help.

6. **Perform CPR.** If one of your companions is having a heart attack and becomes unresponsive and stops breathing, perform CPR.

CPR (CARDIOPULMONARY RESUSCITATION)

IS IT A HEART ATTACK?

Heart attacks are one of those emergencies that are easily recognizable on TV — the numb arm, the dramatic clutching of the chest. But determining if you're having a heart attack in real life can be another matter. Pain may come on suddenly or gradually, with exertion or at rest.

A heart attack may cause one or more of the following signs and symptoms:

+ Chest pain, at times intense or prolonged, that's often described as heavy pressure, squeezing or fullness under the breast-bone or a weight upon the chest
+ Pain that extends beyond your chest, radiating to a shoulder, one or both arms, the back, and even your neck, jaw and teeth
+ Pain in the upper abdomen that feels like severe indigestion
+ Nausea, with or without vomiting
+ Shortness of breath with or without chest discomfort
+ Breaking out in a cold sweat
+ Weakness or lightheadedness
+ Restlessness and anxiety

SEVERE ASTHMA ATTACK

Does your friend seem to be huffing and puffing up that hill with more trouble than usual? Do you hear wheezing as you walk long distances? People with asthma may experience occasional or even frequent asthma attacks. Often a person's asthma-rescue medication is all that's needed to improve symptoms. Occasionally, more serious or even life-threatening asthma attacks may occur.

SIGNS AND SYMPTOMS » ASTHMA ATTACK

+ Severe shortness of breath
+ Chest tightness or pain
+ Coughing or wheezing
+ Rapid breathing
+ Inability to speak more than short phrases
+ Severe anxiety
+ A rapid pulse
+ Excessive sweating
+ A bluish cast to the person's face and lips

TREATMENT » ASTHMA ATTACK

1. **Assess the situation.** Establish that the problem isn't a choking emergency.
2. **Seek emergency care.** Call 911 or activate the SOS button on an emergency device.

 PAGE 146

146

3. **Help with inhaler use.** If the person has a quick-acting (rescue) inhaler, help them use it.
4. **Keep calm.** Keep the person calm, comfortable and sitting upright.
5. **Perform CPR.** If the person becomes unresponsive or stops breathing, begin CPR.

DROWNING

If you find an individual struggling or submerged in water and you believe you're strong enough and sufficiently trained to rescue the person, do so immediately. If you're not a strong swimmer or not sure you can manage the person by yourself, get help. Remember that many people remain silent and are relatively still while drowning, which means individuals might be in danger even if they're not shouting for help or flailing.

TREATMENT » DROWNING

1. **Check for hazards.** Throughout rescue and treatment, make sure your safety isn't compromised.
2. **Once the person has been rescued, check for breathing.** If the person isn't breathing and is unresponsive, begin CPR.
3. **If you're not alone, have someone get help while you provide care.** Call 911 if you're within

cell range or activate the SOS button on an emergency device.

4. **Immediately begin to breathe for the person if they aren't breathing.** Don't waste time trying to drain the person's lungs of water. Air should still reach the lungs despite any residual water. Clear the airway of any debris and deliver two quick breaths. Continue to breathe for the person every few seconds while moving them to shore or a boat.

5. **Get medical attention.** Drowning can result in various medical complications, so seek emergency medical care even after a successful rescue.

DROWNING PREVENTION

Drowning can happen to anyone. To prevent a panicky scenario, take these measures:

+ Learn how to swim.
+ Supervise children when they're in or near water.
+ Learn CPR.
+ Check the forecast.
+ Learn about water risks in the area you plan to visit. Sneaky currents, flash-flood danger, hidden rocks and hazardous waves can increase the risk of drowning.
+ Don't drink alcohol before or during water activities, since it impairs judgment and coordination.
+ Always swim or boat with a buddy.

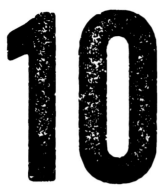

10
PHYSICAL TRAUMA

A traumatic injury is a sudden injury that can threaten life or limb and includes musculoskeletal injuries, such as broken bones, joint dislocations and amputations, and facial injuries, such as tooth loss and eye injuries. A traumatic wound can also result from blunt force trauma, such as a severe blow to the head from a falling rock or injuries from falling off a cliff. Usually, these kinds of injuries require professional medical care. But in a remote setting, it's a good idea to know how to respond until help arrives.

SPRAINS

Watch out for that exposed root or ankle-rolling rock on the trail. The National Institutes of Health reports that 70% of non-fatal injuries in the wilderness are broken bones and sprains, most commonly from a twisted ankle. A sprain occurs when a violent twist or stretch injures or tears the ligaments attached to bone.

If a popping sound and immediate difficulty using the joint accompany the injury, this could indicate a fracture or sprain.

Accidents that cause sprains can also cause serious injuries, including fractures. Seek medical help if your sprain doesn't improve after two or three days.

Get emergency medical assistance if:

+ You're unable to bear weight on the injured leg, the joint feels unstable or numb, or you can't move the joint. This may mean the ligament was completely torn or the bone is broken. On the way to a doctor, apply a cold pack.
+ You develop redness or red streaks that spread out from the injured area. This may mean you have an infection.
+ You have pain directly over the bones of an injured joint.
+ You have a severe sprain or broken bones. Inadequate or delayed treatment of severe sprains or broken bones may contribute to long-term joint instability.

Ankle sprains are the most common type of sprain. Wrist, knee and thumb sprains are also common. Sprained ligaments often swell rapidly and are painful. Generally, the greater the pain and swelling, the more severe the injury. For minor sprains, you can treat the injury yourself with Rest, Ice, Compression and Elevation (R.I.C.E.).

SIGNS AND SYMPTOMS » SPRAINS

+ Pain and tenderness in the affected area.
+ Rapid swelling, sometimes accompanied by mild bruising.
+ Impaired joint function.

1. **Rest the injured limb.** Don't avoid all activity but rest the affected limb. If a leg or ankle is injured, increase activity and weight-bearing slowly, as tolerated. A splint or brace also may be helpful.

2. **Ice the area.** Use a cold pack, a slush bath or a compression sleeve filled with cold water to help limit swelling after an injury. Try to ice the area as soon as possible after the injury and continue to ice it for 15 to 20 minutes, at least four times a day, for the first 48 hours or until swelling improves. Don't use ice for too long or apply it directly to the skin, as this can cause tissue damage.

3. **Compress the area with an elastic wrap or bandage.** If you don't have ice, soak the dressing in a cool body of water, if there's one nearby. Compressive wraps or sleeves made from elastic or neoprene are best. Compress the area — not so tight that the pressure cuts off blood supply, but tight enough that the joint feels supported.

4. **Elevate the injured limb above your heart whenever possible.** This helps to limit swelling.

Sprains can take days to months to recover. As the pain and swelling improve, gently begin using the injured area. You should feel a gradual, progressive improvement.

FRACTURES

A fracture is a broken bone. It requires medical attention. If the broken bone is the result of major trauma or injury, call 911 if you're within cell range or activate the SOS button on an emergency device. If you suspect a fracture, protect the injured area from further damage. Don't try to align the broken bone. Call for emergency help if:

+ The person is unresponsive, isn't breathing or isn't moving. Begin CPR if there's no breathing or heartbeat.
+ There's heavy bleeding.
+ Even gentle pressure or movement causes pain.
+ The limb or joint appears deformed.
+ The bone has pierced the skin.
+ The injured limb is numb or tingly, or the fingers or toes have a bluish hue.
+ You suspect a bone is broken in the neck, head or back.

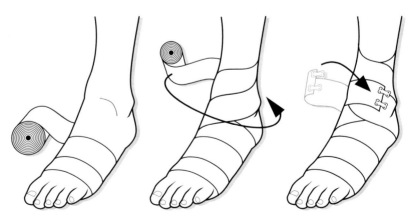

The correct method of wrapping a sprained ankle.

+ Swelling or bruising over a bone
+ Deformity of the affected limb
+ Localized pain that gets worse when the injured area is moved or pressure is put on it
+ Loss of function at the fracture site
+ A broken bone protruding from the skin

TREATMENT » FRACTURES

Take these actions immediately while waiting for medical help:

1. **Don't move the person except if necessary to avoid further injury.**

2. **Check for a pulse below the fracture.** Make sure the wound is between the person's heart and the place where you're checking for the pulse (see page 175). If there's no pulse, blood may not be flowing past the injury and the person is at risk of losing the fractured limb.

3. **Stop the bleeding.** If there's a cut on top of a fracture, apply pressure directly on the wound with a sterile bandage or even a piece of clean clothing to stop the bleeding. If nothing else is available, use your hand, but don't injure yourself on sharp bone fragments. Maintain pressure until the bleeding stops. If possible, elevate the site of the fracture to reduce blood flow.

PAGE 154

4. **Immobilize the injured area.** Don't try to realign the bone or push a bone that's sticking out back into place. Apply a splint to the area above and below the fracture sites. Padding the splints can help reduce discomfort.

5. **Apply ice to limit swelling and relieve the pain.** Don't apply ice directly to the skin. Wrap the ice in a towel, cloth or some other material before placing it on the injured area. Soak the dressing in a cool body of water if no ice is available.

6. **Treat for shock.** If the person is faint, pale or breathing with short, rapid breaths, treat them for shock. Lay the person down with the head slightly lower than the body and, if possible, elevate the legs.

SPLINTING OR IMMOBILIZING FRACTURES

Splints can be fashioned out of any rigid material, such as hiking sticks or poles, wood (branches), skis and paddles. How to splint the fracture depends on the location of the break. A spinal injury or hip or pelvic fracture can't be splinted and must be immobilized in another way.

PHYSICAL TRAUMA

1. **Pad the splint with gauze or cloth, then apply it to the injured limb.** The splint should be longer than the bone it's splinting and extend below and above the injury.
2. **Fasten the splint to the limb with gauze or strips of cloth, tape or other material.** Splint the limb firmly to prevent motion but not so tightly that blood flow is stopped.
   » A simple splint that works well is to put one or more pillows around the limb and tape across the pillows.

Immobilizing arm fractures

Place a broken arm in a sling. You can make a sling from a large piece of cloth or a sheet if needed (see page 156). Place a swathe-wrap over the sling to keep the arm close to the body. Immobilizing the arm helps prevent the broken bones from moving and reduces pain.

Immobilizing leg fractures

If a lower part of the leg is broken, place the entire leg between two splints. See the illustration on page 159. Another option is to place padding around the leg and tape across the padding. A broken thighbone requires that the hip joint also be immobilized.

Fashioning a sling

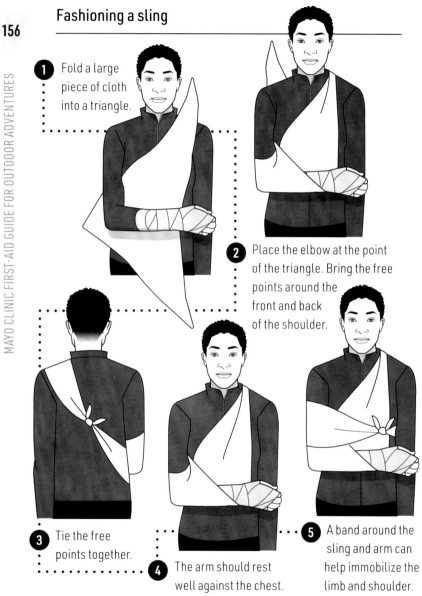

1 Fold a large piece of cloth into a triangle.

2 Place the elbow at the point of the triangle. Bring the free points around the front and back of the shoulder.

3 Tie the free points together.

4 The arm should rest well against the chest.

5 A band around the sling and arm can help immobilize the limb and shoulder.

HIP OR PELVIC FRACTURES

Hip or pelvic fractures are usually caused by falls or other accidents. Suspect a broken pelvis or hip in case of:

+ Pain in the hip, lower back or groin area.
+ Pain in these areas that worsens with movement of one or both legs.
+ An inability to walk or pain when bearing weight.

TREATMENT » HIP OR PELVIC FRACTURES

1. **Get emergency medical attention.** Call 911 if you're within cell range or activate the SOS button on an emergency device.
2. **Don't move the person.** If you need to move the person, gently reposition them on a board or flat surface. Don't try to straighten an injured leg or hip that seems oddly positioned.

DISLOCATIONS

A dislocation is an injury in which two bones are forced from their normal positions and come apart. Dislocation usually involves the body's larger joints and results from trauma, such as falling. In adults, the most common site of injury is the shoulder. In children, it's the elbow. Your thumb and fingers are also vulnerable if forcibly bent the wrong way.

General signs and symptoms of a dislocation can include sudden and severe pain swelling, a joint that's out of position, misshapen and difficult to move, and a feeling of instability.

SIGNS AND SYMPTOMS » DISLOCATED KNEECAP

+ Swelling
+ A popping sensation while the kneecap falls out of the joint, followed by an inability to move the knee
+ Severe knee pain
+ Inability to straighten the knee
+ Inability to walk
+ A deformity (The kneecap sits to the side of where it should be.)

If the kneecap is dislocated, gently straightening the leg will often cause the kneecap to slide back into place.

SIGNS AND SYMPTOMS » DISLOCATED SHOULDER

+ A visibly deformed or out-of-place shoulder
+ Swelling or bruising
+ Pain; the muscles in the shoulder might spasm, which can increase the pain
+ Inability to move the shoulder
+ Numbness, weakness or tingling near the injury, such as down the arm

Leg splints

If a lower part of the leg is broken, place the entire leg between two splints. A broken thighbone requires that the hip joint also be immobilized.

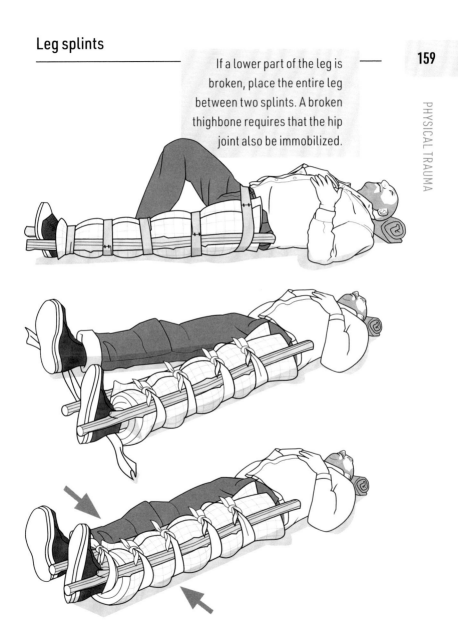

Other than the kneecap, dislocated joints shouldn't be put back in place. This can damage the joint and its surrounding muscles, ligaments, nerves or blood vessels. Also, putting the bones back in place often requires sedation. In case of a dislocated kneecap, sometimes the kneecap may slide back into place on its own, but it's still important to seek medical attention to ensure other structures in the knee are correctly aligned and not damaged.

TREATMENT » DISLOCATIONS

While waiting for medical attention:

1. **Remove jewelry.** Immediately remove any jewelry from an injured finger or toe, if possible.
2. **Splint the joint in the position it's in.** In the case of a shoulder dislocation, use a sling.
3. **Ice the injured joint.** Apply ice to the joint, if possible, to help reduce pain and swelling.
4. **Take pain medication.** To help reduce pain, take an over-the-counter pain reliever.

EYE INJURIES

Eye injuries should be taken seriously because complications can impair vision. Potential traumatic injuries to the eye include corneal abrasions, blood in an eye, a black eye and eyelid lacerations. Many eye injuries and illnesses can be prevented with protective eyewear and good handwashing before touching the eyes.

CORNEAL ABRASION (SCRATCH)

Most eye injuries affect the cornea — the clear, protective "window" at the front of the eye. A speck of sand, dust, dirt, plant matter or even a contact lens that's worn for too long can scratch the cornea, causing a corneal abrasion.

Because the cornea is extremely sensitive, abrasions can be very painful. Instantaneous pain at the moment of injury followed by persistent pain, tearing up and redness are key indications of a corneal abrasion. Some abrasions can become infected and result in a corneal ulcer, which is a serious problem.

SIGNS AND SYMPTOMS » CORNEAL ABRASION

+ Pain
+ Blurry vision
+ A gritty feeling in the eye
+ Tearing
+ Redness
+ Sensitivity to light
+ Headache

TREATMENT » CORNEAL ABRASION

1. **Rinse your eye with clean water or a saline solution.** You can use an eyecup or a small, clean drinking glass positioned with its rim resting on the bone at the base of your eye

 PAGE 162

socket (see page 117). Rinsing the eye may wash out a foreign object. Blink several times. This movement may remove small particles.

2. **Pull the upper eyelid over the lower eyelid.** This may cause your eye to tear, which may help wash out the particle.

Use the following tips to avoid making the injury worse:

+ Don't try to remove an object that's embedded in your eye or makes your eye difficult to close. Tape some gauze over the eye and seek immediate medical attention.

+ Don't rub your eye after an injury.

+ Don't touch your eye with cotton swabs, tweezers or other instruments.

+ If you use contact lenses, don't wear them while your eye is healing.

Most corneal abrasions heal in a few days but should be treated with antibiotic drops or ointment to reduce the risk of infection.

BLOOD IN THE EYE

Bleeding in the whites of the eyes can occur for a number of reasons, like powerful coughing, sneezing or vomiting, especially in people who travel to high altitudes. Though unsettling to look at, if your vision isn't affected, it's OK to continue your outdoor activities with blood in the eye.

Immediately descend if the issue affects your vision or you notice other signs of altitude sickness. Blood in the eye also can result from trauma, such as a blow to the eye or an injury that perforates the eye. Seek immediate medical care.

BLACK EYE

A black eye is caused by bleeding beneath the skin around the eye. Most injuries that cause a black eye aren't serious. But a black eye could be a sign of a more concerning injury, such as an internal injury to the eye or a fracture of the thin bones around the eye. You may have a skull fracture if you have double vision, bruising around both eyes (raccoon eyes), bleeding from the nose, or tenderness to the bones around the eyes.

TREATMENT » BLACK EYE

1. **Apply a cold compress soon after the injury.** Place a cold pack or cloth filled with ice to the area around the eye. Take care not to press on the eye itself. Applying cold will reduce swelling. Repeat several times a day for a day or two.
2. **Seek medical care.** If you see blood in the white or colored parts of the eye or have vision problems, such as double vision or blurring,

PAGE 164

seek immediate care. Also seek care if you have severe pain or bruising around both eyes, or bleeding in an eye or from the nose.

3. **Apply warm or hot compresses.** This may be helpful after a few days when the swelling has gone down. Repeat several times a day for a day or two.

EYELID LACERATION

If an eyelid is cut, apply clean gauze to the eye without applying pressure and seek immediate medical care.

DENTAL INJURIES

When a permanent tooth is accidentally knocked out in one piece, it can sometimes be reimplanted, so be sure to save the tooth and seek medical attention as quickly as possible. If reimplantation doesn't occur within two hours after the tooth is knocked out — sooner is better — the likelihood of success becomes poor. So it's vital to get emergency dental care.

TREATMENT » TOOTH LOSS

1. **Handle the tooth by the top or crown only.** Don't touch the roots.
2. **Inspect the crown and root.** Determine if any portion of either seems to be missing or fractured.

3. **Don't rub or scrape the tooth to remove debris.** This damages the root surface, making the tooth less likely to survive.

    »   If the tooth has dirt or foreign material on it, gently rinse the tooth briefly — no more than 10 seconds — in a bowl of clean, luke-warm water to remove the debris. Don't hold it under running water, because too much tap water could kill the cells on the root surface that help reattach the tooth.

4. **Try to put your tooth back in the socket.** If it doesn't go all the way into place, bite down slowly and gently on gauze or a moistened paper towel. Hold the tooth in place until you see a dentist or a doctor.

    »   If you can't put your tooth back in the socket, place it between your cheek and gum, in a container with cold milk or in your own saliva.

SPINAL INJURIES

If you suspect a back or neck (spinal) injury, don't move the injured person. Permanent paralysis and other serious complications can result from moving a person with a spinal injury. Broken bones around the spine can move and damage the spinal cord so keep the person flat and move them as little as possible.

Assume a person has a spinal injury if:

+ There's evidence of a head injury that may include a skull fracture.
+ There's an ongoing change in the person's consciousness.
+ The person complains of pain in the neck or back.
+ An injury has exerted substantial force on the back or head.
+ The person complains of weakness, numbness, or paralysis or lacks control of their limbs, bladder or bowels.
+ The neck or body is twisted or positioned oddly.

TREATMENT » SUSPECTED SPINAL INJURY

1. **Seek emergency medical care.** Call 911 if you're within cell range or activate the SOS button on an emergency device.
2. **Keep the person still.** Place heavy towels or rolled cloth on both sides of the neck or hold the head and neck to prevent movement.
3. **Avoid moving the head and neck.** Provide as much first aid as possible without moving the person's head or neck. If you must move the person because of choking or immediate danger, use at least two people and try to keep the person's head, neck and back carefully aligned.
4. **If the person shows no signs of circulation (breathing, coughing or movement), begin CPR.** Don't tilt the head back to open the airway. Use your fingers to gently grasp the jaw and lift it

forward. If the person has no pulse, begin chest compressions.
5. **Keep helmet on.** If the person is wearing a helmet, don't remove it.

HEAD INJURIES

Most head injuries are minor because the skull provides considerable protection to the brain. Sometimes, though, a blow to the head can cause injuries that require attention. Any of the following symptoms may indicate a serious head injury:

SIGNS AND SYMPTOMS » SERIOUS HEAD INJURY

+ Severe bleeding from the head or face
+ Bleeding or fluid leakage from the nose or ears
+ Vomiting
+ Severe headache
+ Change in consciousness for more than a few seconds
+ Discoloration below the eyes or behind the ears
+ Not breathing
+ Confusion or agitation
+ Loss of balance
+ Weakness or an inability to use an arm or leg
+ Unequal pupil size
+ Slurred speech
+ Seizures

1. **Seek emergency medical attention.** Call 911 if you're within cell range or activate the SOS button on an emergency device.
2. **Keep the person still.** Until medical help arrives, keep the injured person lying down and quiet. For a severe head injury, assume the spine may be injured as well. Don't move the person unless necessary. Avoid moving the person's neck. If the person is wearing a helmet, don't remove it.
3. **Stop any bleeding.** Apply firm pressure to the bleeding wound with sterile gauze or a clean cloth. Don't apply direct pressure to the wound if you suspect a skull fracture.
4. **Watch for changes in breathing and alertness.** If the person shows no signs of circulation — no breathing, coughing or movement — begin CPR.

CONCUSSION

Concussions are usually caused by a blow to the head or violent shaking of the head and upper body. Some concussions cause you to lose consciousness, but most don't. Signs and symptoms of a concussion can be subtle and may not show up immediately. They can last for days, weeks or even longer. Common symptoms are headache, loss of memory (amnesia) and confusion.

Any head trauma that produces concussion symptoms needs to be evaluated by a medical professional. Seek

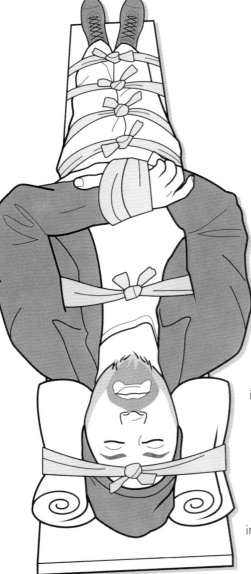

Neck and back injuries require special precautions. If medical help is unavailable and the injured person must be moved, recruit several people to help. Neck and back injuries can lead to permanent paralysis. Proper use of a backboard immobilizes the victim's head, neck and spine.

emergency care for anyone who sustains a head injury with signs and symptoms such as the following:

+ Repeated vomiting or nausea
+ A loss of consciousness lasting longer than 30 seconds
+ A headache that gets worse over time
+ Fluid or blood draining from the nose or ears
+ Vision or eye disturbances, such as pupils that are bigger than normal (dilated pupils) or pupils of unequal sizes
+ Ringing in the ears that doesn't go away
+ Weakness in the arms or legs
+ Changes in behavior
+ Confusion or disorientation, such as difficulty recognizing people or places
+ Slurred speech or other changes in speech
+ Obvious difficulty with mental function
+ Changes in coordination, such as stumbling or clumsiness
+ Seizures or convulsions
+ Persistent or recurrent dizziness
+ Symptoms that worsen over time
+ Large head bumps or bruises on the head

TREATMENT » CONCUSSION

1. **Have the person rest.** Limit activities that require physical or mental exertion.
2. **Monitor symptoms.** The first night after the injury, wake the person every few hours. If the person becomes confused or vomits more than two times, seek immediate medical attention.

INTRACRANIAL HEMATOMA

An intracranial hematoma results when a blood vessel — an artery or vein — ruptures between the skull and brain. Leaking blood accumulates inside the skull (hematoma) and presses on the brain tissue.

The most common cause of an intracranial hematoma is trauma, such as a strong blow to the head or a fall. Signs and symptoms may develop right after a head injury, or they may take hours to appear.

SIGNS AND SYMPTOMS » INTRACRANIAL HEMATOMA

+ Headache that gets worse
+ Vomiting
+ Dizziness
+ Unequal pupil size

An intracranial hematoma can be life-threatening, requiring emergency treatment. Seek emergency care if the injured person:
+ Is drowsy and progressively loses consciousness.
+ Has a persistent headache.
+ Experiences vomiting, blurred vision or unsteadiness.
+ Has pupils that are unequal in size.
+ Slurs their speech.
+ Has loss of movement (paralysis) on the opposite side of the body from the head injury.
+ Experiences confusion.
+ Is lethargic.
+ Has one or more seizures.

If you don't notice signs and symptoms right after the head injury, watch for physical, mental and emotional changes. For example, if someone seems fine after a head injury but later becomes confused or lethargic, seek immediate medical care. If you hit your own head, even if you initially feel fine, ask someone to watch out for you.

SKULL FRACTURES

Visible bone fragments or brain matter are obvious signs of a skull fracture. A fracture also may produce other, less noticeable signs and symptoms.

SIGNS AND SYMPTOMS » SKULL FRACTURES

+ Bruising or discoloration behind the ear or around the eyes
+ Blood or watery fluid leaking from the ears or nose
+ Pupils of unequal size, accompanied by a change in mental status, such as confusion or unconsciousness
+ Deformity of the skull, including swelling or depressions

TREATMENT » SKULL FRACTURE

A skull fracture is a medical emergency and must be treated promptly to avoid brain damage and even death.

1. **Seek medical attention.** Call 911 if you're within cell range or activate the SOS button on an emergency device.

2. **Keep the person still.** The injured person should lie down with their head and shoulders slightly elevated. Don't move the person unless necessary, and avoid moving the person's neck.

3. **Don't apply pressure.** Don't apply direct pressure to the wound if you suspect a skull fracture. Treat any bleeding by gently holding some clean gauze to the area.

4. **Watch for changes in breathing and alertness.** If the person shows no signs of circulation — no breathing, coughing or movement — begin CPR.

AMPUTATION

When a finger, toe or larger body part is severed, risks include significant blood loss, shock and infection. They can be life-threatening. Seek emergency help as quickly as you can, getting both the injured person and the severed part to a hospital, where the part may possibly be reattached. Until help arrives:

TREATMENT » AMPUTATION

1. **Stop the bleeding.** The first goal of emergency treatment is to stop blood loss. Apply pressure to the wound with a sterile bandage or clean cloth.

2. **Have the person lie down, if possible.** The limb with the injury should be slightly elevated.

PAGE 174

3. **Wrap the wound.** When the bleeding is under control, wrap the wound with additional layers.

4. **Apply a tourniquet.** If bleeding continues, application of a tourniquet may be necessary (see page 78).

5. **Check for other injuries.** Once you have the bleeding under control, examine the person for other signs of injury you may not have noticed.

6. **Save the severed part.** Once the person is stable, carefully put the amputated body part in a clean plastic bag or wrap it in a clean cloth. Keep the severed part cold, if possible.

CHECKING A PULSE

You can check for a person's pulse on their wrist, ankle or neck.

+ **Wrist.** Turn the person's hand so that the palm is facing up. With your other hand, gently place two of your fingertips on the groove just below the fold of the wrist and in the groove next to the tendon, about an inch below the thumb. Apply enough pressure to feel each beat.

+ **Ankle.** Apply several fingers just behind the inner part of the ankle.

+ **Neck.** Place your index and middle fingers on the side of the person's neck, in the hollow area just beside their windpipe.

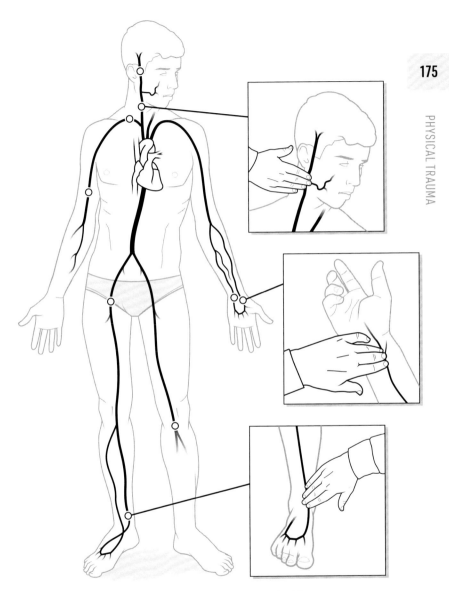

Where to check for a pulse on the neck, wrist and ankle.
The circles indicate other arterial pressure points.

SHOCK

Shock is a critical condition brought on by the sudden drop in blood flow through the body. Shock may result from trauma, heatstroke, blood loss or an allergic reaction. It also may result from severe infection, poisoning, severe burns or a variety of other causes. When a person is in shock, their organs don't get enough blood or oxygen. Seek emergency medical attention. If shock isn't treated, it can lead to permanent organ damage or even death.

SIGNS AND SYMPTOMS » SHOCK

+ Cool, clammy skin
+ Pale or ashen skin
+ A gray or bluish tinge to lips or fingernails
+ Rapid pulse
+ Rapid breathing
+ Dizziness or fainting
+ Weakness or fatigue
+ Changes in mental status, like lethargy or sleepiness
+ Changes in behavior, such as anxiety or agitation

1. Lay the person down and elevate their legs, unless you think this may cause pain or further injury.
2. Keep the person still and don't move them unless necessary.
3. Begin CPR if the person shows no signs of life.
4. Loosen tight clothing and cover the person with a blanket.
5. Don't let the person eat or drink anything.
6. If the person vomits or is bleeding from the mouth, and no spinal injury is suspected, turn the person onto their side to prevent choking.

To avoid or reduce the effects of shock, keep the person warm and elevate the legs and feet above the level of the heart. This will maximize the flow of blood to the head.

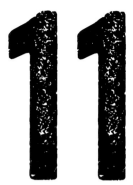

11

FAINTING, SEIZURE AND STROKE

udden loss of consciousness is an alarming medical event that may occur for several reasons. Basic fainting spells are the least serious. For example, some perfectly healthy people faint at the sight of blood and recover completely in a matter of minutes. But it's important not to ignore fainting or seizures, as they can be a sign of something serious. When someone passes out and doesn't immediately recover, or has a seizure, seek immediate medical care.

FAINTING

Fainting occurs when the brain doesn't receive enough blood for a brief time. This causes a loss of consciousness, which is usually regained quickly. Often, it's the fall during a fainting spell that causes the most serious injury. Fainting may have no medical significance. Or the cause may be a serious disorder, possibly involving the heart. Therefore, treat loss of consciousness as a serious medical condition until the symptoms are relieved and the cause is known.

TREATMENT » IF YOU FEEL FAINT

1. **Lie or sit down.** To reduce the chance of fainting again, don't get up too quickly.
2. **Lower your head.** Place your head between your knees if you sit down.

TREATMENT » IF SOMEONE ELSE FAINTS

1. **Position the person on their back.** If there are no injuries and the person is breathing, raise their legs above heart level, if possible. Loosen belts, collars or other tight clothing.
2. **Don't let the person get up too fast.** This will reduce the chance of fainting again.
3. **Seek emergency help.** If the person doesn't regain consciousness within one minute, call 911 if you're within cell range or activate the SOS button on an emergency device.
4. **Check for breathing.** Check for a pulse and to see if the person is breathing. If the person isn't breathing, begin CPR. Seek emergency medical assistance and continue CPR until help arrives or the person begins to breathe.
5. **Control bleeding with direct pressure.** If the person was injured in a fall associated with fainting, treat bumps, bruises or cuts appropriately.

SEIZURE

A seizure is a sudden, uncontrolled burst of electrical activity in the brain. It can cause changes in behavior, movements and levels of consciousness. There are many types of seizures, with a range of symptoms and severity. Most seizures last from 30 seconds to 2 minutes. A seizure that lasts longer than five minutes is a medical emergency. Seizures can happen after a stroke or head injury. They also may be caused by a high fever, an infection, another illness, or alcohol or drug misuse. Many times, the cause is unknown.

SIGNS AND SYMPTOMS » SEIZURE

Symptoms vary based on the type of seizure and can range from mild to severe. Seizure signs and symptoms may include the following:

+ Temporary confusion
+ A staring spell
+ Jerking movements of the arms and legs that can't be controlled
+ Loss of consciousness or awareness

1. **Keep the person from injuring themself.** If vomiting occurs, try to turn the person's head so that the vomit is expelled and isn't breathed in (aspirated) to the windpipe or lungs. Clear the area around the person to reduce their risk of injury during uncontrolled body movements. Although the person may briefly stop breathing — and may turn bluish from lack of oxygen — breathing almost always returns without the need for CPR.

2. **Position the person on their side.** Once the seizure is over, roll the person onto their side. This allows for normal breathing and allows fluids such as vomit or blood to be expelled.

3. **Monitor cognitive function.** After the seizure, the person may be confused for a while. Watch the person until their mental function returns completely.

4. **Seek emergency medical care.** Get immediate help if someone is having a seizure and any of the following occurs:
   » The seizure lasts more than five minutes.
   » The person isn't breathing after the seizure stops.
   » A second seizure follows immediately.
   » The seizure is accompanied by a high fever.
   » The seizure is accompanied by heat exhaustion.

» The person who had the seizure is pregnant.
» The person who had the seizure has diabetes.
» The seizure resulted in an injury.
» This was the first time the person had a seizure.

5. **Treat injuries.** Care for any injuries resulting from a fall during a seizure.

STROKE

A stroke happens when there's bleeding into the brain or when blood flow to the brain is blocked. When brain cells are deprived of essential nutrients, they start dying within minutes. Seek immediate medical help. A stroke is a true emergency. The earlier the person receives treatment, the greater the chance of keeping damage to a minimum.

Signs and symptoms of a stroke may last only a few minutes, or they may persist for several hours. All warning signs, even short-term ones, should be taken seriously.

SIGNS AND SYMPTOMS » STROKE

+ **Trouble speaking and understanding what others are saying.** The person may experience confusion, slur their words or have difficulty understanding speech.
+ **Paralysis or numbness of the face, arm or leg.** This

often affects just one side of the body. To help determine if the person is having a stroke, follow the instructions for F.A.S.T. on the next page.

+ **Problems seeing in one or both eyes.** The person may suddenly have blurred or blackened vision in one or both eyes, or see double.

+ **Headache.** A sudden, severe headache, possibly accompanied by vomiting, dizziness or altered consciousness, may indicate a stroke.

+ **Trouble walking.** The person may stumble or lose their balance, or they may experience sudden dizziness or a loss of coordination.

TREATMENT » STROKE

Seek immediate medical attention if you notice any signs or symptoms of a stroke, even if they seem to come and go or they disappear completely. If you're with someone you suspect is having a stroke, watch the person carefully while waiting for help.

1. **Seek emergency medical assistance.** Call 911 if you're within cell range or activate the SOS button on an emergency device.

2. **Monitor breathing.** While waiting for emergency medical help, pay attention to the person's breathing.

   » If breathing stops, begin CPR.

3. **Watch for vomiting.** If vomiting occurs, turn

the person on their side so they don't choke.
Don't allow the person to eat or drink anything.

4. **Protect from further injury.** If paralysis is
    present, protect the paralyzed limbs from injury
    that might occur when the person moves about
    or is transported.

**THINK
F.A.S.T.**

If you think a person may be having a stroke,
use the F.A.S.T. acronym as a response tool:

+ **Face.** Ask the person to smile. Does one
  side of the face droop?

+ **Arm.** Ask the person to raise both arms.
  Does one arm drift downward? Or is one
  arm unable to rise?

+ **Speech.** Ask the person to repeat a simple
  sentence, such as "The sky is blue." Is the
  speech slurred? Can the person repeat the
  sentence correctly?

+ **Time.** If you observe any of these signs,
  seek medical help immediately. Don't
  wait to see if symptoms stop — every
  minute counts. Try to determine when
  the signs and symptoms began so you
  can tell medical personnel when you
  first noticed something was wrong.
  This helps guide treatment.

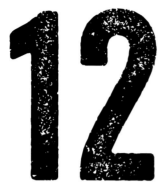

12

COLD-RELATED EMERGENCIES

eather can change quickly. If you're ill-prepared, unexpected hail, snow, wind or rain can turn an adventure into a shivering — even dangerous — ordeal. Overexposure to cold and damp weather can lead to frostbite or hypothermia. Proper attire and acclimatization are the best ways to boost morale while managing the cold.

COLD-WEATHER PREPAREDNESS

You can do several things to reduce risk of injury from frostbite and hypothermia:

+ **Stay dry.** Your body loses heat faster when the skin is wet.
+ **Protect yourself from wind.** Exposed skin is especially vulnerable and can freeze in minutes when wind combines with subfreezing temperatures.
    » For example: An outdoor temperature of minus 20 F combined with a 10 mph wind produces a wind chill factor of minus 41 F.
+ **Wear warm clothing.** Choose clothes that both shield against the wind and breathe. Layers of light,

loose-fitting clothes trap air, which adds insulation. The outer layer should be water-repellent and windproof.

+ **Cover your head, neck and face.** Much of your body heat is lost as it rises from the top of your body.
+ **Wear warm socks and mittens.** If you're going to be in subfreezing temperatures for more than a few minutes, wear two layers of socks. In addition, wear mittens, which protect your fingers more effectively than gloves do.
+ **Stay alert to numbness.** If part of your body starts feeling painful or numb, that's a clue your skin is beginning to freeze. Time to rewarm yourself.

FROSTBITE

Frostbite occurs when skin and underlying tissues freeze after being exposed to very cold temperatures. The areas most likely to be affected are the fingertips, toes, earlobes, cheeks, chin and tip of the nose. Anyone can get frostbite, but people with circulatory problems are at greater risk. As with many outdoor injuries, excessive consumption of alcohol or other drugs increases the risk of frostbite.

Early signs and symptoms of frostbite are patches of discolored skin and burning pain. The condition then can progress to skin that's cold, numb, stiff or waxy looking and that may appear white, grayish yellow, brown or ashen, depending on the severity and usual skin color. As the area thaws, the flesh may change color and become very painful. Large, clear or bloody blisters may develop.

1. **Check for hypothermia.** Get emergency medical help if you suspect hypothermia (see page 191).

2. **Protect your skin from further damage.** If there's any chance the affected areas will freeze again, don't thaw them. If they're already thawed, wrap them up so that they don't refreeze.

3. **Warm frostbitten hands by tucking them into your armpits.** Protect your face, nose or ears by covering the area with dry, gloved hands. Don't rub the affected skin with snow or anything else. Don't walk on frostbitten feet or toes, if possible.

4. **Get out of the cold.** Once you're in a warm space, remove wet clothes and wrap up in a warm blanket.

5. **Gently rewarm frostbitten areas.** Soak frostbitten fingers, toes or other extremities in warm water — 105 F to 110 F. If a thermometer isn't available, test the water by placing an uninjured hand or elbow in it — it should feel very warm, not hot. Soak for 20 to 30 minutes or until the skin becomes its normal color or loses its numbness. For the face or ears, apply a warm, wet washcloth. Don't rewarm frostbitten skin with direct heat, such as a stove, heat lamp, fireplace or heating pad.

6. **Drink warm liquids.** Tea, hot chocolate or soup can help warm from the inside. Don't drink alcohol.

7. **Take medication.** If you're in pain, consider an over-the-counter pain reliever.

PAGE 190

8. **Know what to expect as skin thaws.** You'll feel tingling and burning as the skin warms and normal blood flow returns. Take care not to break any blisters that may form on the affected skin.

HYPOTHERMIA

Under most conditions, your body hums along at a steady and healthy temperature. However, when you're exposed to cold, wet environments for long periods of time — particularly if your clothing is damp — the body's temperature-control mechanisms get overwhelmed. When you lose more heat than your body can generate, hypothermia can result. For this reason, if your clothes are wet with sweat from hiking up a mountain, it's important to change clothes when you reach the top. As the temperature cools, especially later in the day, wearing sweaty clothes can increase the risk of hypothermia.

Normal body temperature is around 98.6 F. Hypothermia occurs as your body temperature falls below 95 F. When your body temperature drops, your heart, nervous system and other organs can't work normally. Left untreated, hypothermia can lead to complete failure of your heart and respiratory system and eventually to death.

Someone with hypothermia usually isn't aware of their condition because symptoms often begin gradually. When you're very cold, your thinking can get muddled, making it hard to understand what's happening. This might lead you to take chances that you normally wouldn't.

+ Shivering (This may stop as body temperature drops.)
+ Slurred speech or mumbling
+ Slow, shallow breathing
+ Weak pulse
+ Clumsiness or lack of coordination
+ Drowsiness or very low energy
+ Confusion or memory loss
+ Loss of consciousness

TREATMENT » HYPOTHERMIA

1. **Seek immediate medical attention for anyone who appears to have hypothermia.** Call 911 if you're within cell range or activate the SOS button on an emergency device.

2. **Be gentle.** When you're helping a person with hypothermia, handle them gently. Limit movements to only those that are necessary. Don't massage or rub the person. Excessive, vigorous or jarring movements may trigger cardiac arrest.

3. **Move the person out of the cold.** If going indoors isn't possible, protect the person from the wind, especially around the neck and head. Insulate the individual from the cold ground.

4. **Remove wet clothing.** If the person is wearing wet clothing, remove it. Cut away the clothing, if necessary, to avoid excessive movement.

PAGE 192

192

Replace wet clothing with dry coats or blankets.

5. **If further warming is needed, do so gradually.**

» **Use warm, dry compresses.** Or create a makeshift compress of warm water in a plastic bottle. Apply a compress only to the neck, chest wall or groin. If you use a hot water bottle or a chemical hot pack, first wrap it in a towel before applying.

» **Cover the person with blankets.** Use layers of dry blankets or coats to warm the person. Cover the person's head, leaving only the face exposed.

6. **Provide warm beverages.** If the person is alert and able to swallow, provide warm, sweet, drinks.

7. **Monitor breathing.** Begin CPR if the person shows no signs of life.

CAUTION

+ **Don't attempt to warm the arms and legs.** Heating or massaging the limbs of someone in this condition can stress the heart and lungs.

+ **Don't rewarm the person too quickly.** Don't use a heating lamp or hot bath to warm the person. The extreme heat can damage the skin or, even worse, cause irregular heartbeats that can be severe and even fatal.

+ **Don't give the person alcohol or cigarettes.** Alcohol hinders the rewarming process, and tobacco products interfere with circulation.

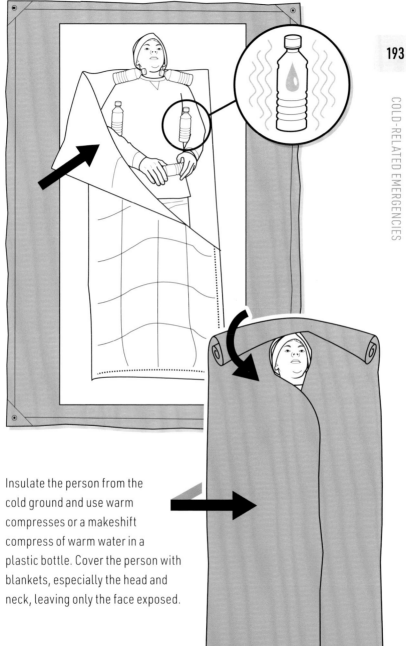

Insulate the person from the cold ground and use warm compresses or a makeshift compress of warm water in a plastic bottle. Cover the person with blankets, especially the head and neck, leaving only the face exposed.

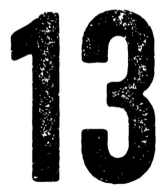

13

HEAT-RELATED EMERGENCIES

lways check the weather before heading out on an adventure, then be sure to pack and dress appropriately. When sun and heat are in the mix, it's important to bring plenty of water, to dress in breathable, protective layers and to wear sunscreen. Without enough shade, water and rest, a sunny romp into the wilderness can turn into a medical emergency.

TO BEAT THE HEAT

+ **Stay out of the sun.** Stay in the shade during the hottest part of the day — usually from noon to 4 p.m.
+ **Limit physical activity.** Reserve vigorous exercise or the most strenuous parts of the hike for early morning or the evening.
+ **Dress for the heat.** Wear clothes that are light colored, lightweight and loose fitting.
+ **Drink lots of liquids.** Avoid excess alcohol and caffeine.
+ **Avoid hot and heavy meals.** Smaller meals combined with healthy snacks are a good idea when the weather gets hot.

PREVENT HEAT-RELATED ILLNESS

Here are some additional tips to avoid heat-related illness during your outdoor activities:

+ **Wear your sun protection.** Apply sunscreen and wear sunglasses and a hat.

+ **Eat salty snacks.** Salty snacks replace the electrolytes your body loses when you sweat. This is especially important when you're being physically active in the heat, which increases how much you sweat.

+ **Rest often, and in the shade, if available.** Take frequent breaks to give your body a rest. Rest under shade to help your body cool off.

+ **Get wet.** Soak a towel or a shirt in water to keep you cool. If water is available, consider completely soaking yourself to keep cool. The water can cool your body and lessen the effects of heat.

+ **Put your backup plan into action.** Use your backup plan if it's too hot to do your planned activity.

+ **Turn back.** Stop and turn around if it gets too hot during your activity.

HEAT STRESS

Under normal conditions, your body's natural control mechanisms help you adjust to the heat. Your body can radiate heat away from itself, and sweating is a very efficient way to cool the body. However, when you're exposed to high temperatures for long periods — especially when there's little breeze and high humidity — your body's normal control mechanisms can get overwhelmed. They can't handle the amount of intense heat bearing down on you, and problems develop.

HEAT EXHAUSTION

Heat exhaustion can occur when your body loses too much water or salt — usually as a result of excessive sweating or dehydration. It can begin suddenly or happen over time, usually after working, exercising or playing in the heat. Heat exhaustion can quickly evolve into heatstroke if steps aren't taken to treat it.

SIGNS AND SYMPTOMS » HEAT EXHAUSTION

+ Heavy sweating
+ Feeling faint
+ Dizziness
+ Fatigue
+ Weak, rapid pulse
+ Feeling dizzy when standing
+ Muscle cramps

+ Nausea or vomiting
+ Headache
+ Mild confusion
+ Decreased urine output

TREATMENT » HEAT EXHAUSTION

1. **Find shelter.** Get the person out of the heat and into the shade or somewhere cool.
2. **Lay the person down and elevate their legs and feet slightly.** If the person is alert, consider wading in a stream to cool down.
3. **Encourage fluids.** Have the person sip chilled water, a drink containing electrolytes or other nonalcoholic beverage without caffeine.
4. **Cool the person.** Mist or sponge the person with cool water.
5. **Monitor the person carefully.**

Seek medical assistance if the person's condition worsens or if the following occurs:
+ Fainting
+ Agitation
+ Confusion
+ Seizures
+ Inability to drink or keep fluids down
+ Core body temperature — measured by rectal thermometer — rises to 104 F (heatstroke)

HEATSTROKE

Heatstroke occurs when your body temperature rises rapidly and you're unable to cool down. It can develop from too much strenuous activity in the heat or by being in a hot place for too long.

Those most at risk are older adults and the very young, as well as people who have experienced previous heat-related illness, have a heart condition, are dehydrated or drink excessive amounts of alcohol. Medications for motion sickness and depression that impair your ability to sweat also can increase heatstroke risk.

SIGNS AND SYMPTOMS » HEATSTROKE

+ Fever of 104 F or greater
+ Hot, dry skin or heavy sweating
+ Nausea and vomiting
+ Flushed skin
+ Rapid pulse
+ Rapid breathing
+ Headache
+ Fainting
+ Changes in mental status or behavior, such as confusion, agitation or slurred speech
+ Seizure
+ Coma

1. **Seek emergency medical care.** Call 911 if you're within cell range or activate the SOS button on an emergency device.
2. **Find shelter.** Move the person out of the heat right away, into a shady or air-conditioned place.
3. **Cool the person by whatever means available.** For example:
    » Put the person in a cool, shallow body of water.
    » Sponge the person with cool water.
    » Mist the person with cool water.
    » Place ice packs or cool wet towels on the neck, armpits and groin.
4. **If the person is conscious, offer chilled water.** Other options include a sports drink containing electrolytes or other nonalcoholic beverage without caffeine.
5. **Begin CPR.** Do this if the person loses consciousness and shows no signs of circulation, such as breathing, coughing or movement.

HEAT CRAMPS

Heat cramps are painful muscle spasms that usually occur during exertion in hot environments. Fluid and electrolyte loss often contributes to heat cramps. The muscles most often affected are large muscle groups, including those in your calves, arms, abdominal wall and back. But heat cramps can develop in any muscle group.

TREATMENT » HEAT CRAMPS

1. Rest briefly and cool down.
2. Drink clear juice or an electrolyte-containing sports drink.
3. Practice gentle, range-of-motion stretching and gentle massage of the affected muscle group.
4. Don't resume strenuous activity for several hours or longer after heat cramps go away.

Seek medical care if the cramps don't go away within an hour or so.

DID YOU KNOW...

Risk of heat-related illness increases with:

+ **High humidity.** It doesn't allow sweat to evaporate as quickly, preventing the body from releasing heat quickly.
+ **High elevation.** It increases your chances of getting dehydrated and sunburned, both of which limit the body's ability to cool down.
+ **Strenuous activities.** Participating in strenuous physical activities, such as hiking or biking, in hot weather can make it difficult for your body to cool off.

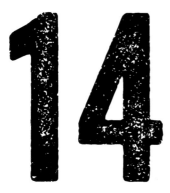

14

INTOXICATION EMERGENCIES

any over-the-counter and prescription medications can have serious consequences when mixed with alcohol or illicit drugs. That's why it's important to take only the recommended or prescribed dose, to abstain from alcohol while on medications and to avoid illegal substances.

ALCOHOL INTOXICATION

Alcohol depresses your central nervous system by acting as a sedative. Alcohol intoxication results as the amount of alcohol in your bloodstream increases. The higher the blood alcohol concentration, the more likely you are to experience bad effects. Initially, alcohol may cause you to feel like you have increased energy. But as you continue to drink, you become drowsy and have less control over your actions.

+ Slurred speech
+ Poor coordination
+ Inappropriate behavior
+ Unstable mood
+ Poor judgment
+ Vomiting
+ Problems with attention or memory
+ Lethargy
+ Unconsciousness

TREATMENT » ALCOHOL INTOXICATION

If you're trying to help someone who's intoxicated:

1. **Stay calm.** Ask the person whether they've taken any medications while drinking. Mixing alcohol with certain drugs can cause the person's condition to quickly deteriorate and become life-threatening.

2. **Prevent aspiration.** If the person vomits, try to prevent them from inhaling (aspirating) vomit into the lungs. Bend their head between their knees, or if the person is lying down, turn their head to one side.

WHEN IT'S AN EMERGENCY

Certain signs and symptoms that accompany heavy drinking may indicate alcohol poisoning — a life-threatening emergency. Seek emergency medical care if a person who's been drinking shows or experiences any of the following:

+ Confusion
+ Vomiting
+ Seizures
+ Slow breathing (fewer than eight breaths per minute)
+ Irregular breathing (a gap of more than 10 seconds between breaths)
+ Blue-tinged skin or pale skin
+ Low body temperature (hypothermia)
+ Difficulty remaining conscious
+ Unconsciousness and can't be awakened
+ Consumption of excessive amounts of alcohol along with other drugs

A person who's unconscious and can't be awakened is at risk of dying. If you suspect that someone has alcohol poisoning — even if you don't see the classic signs and symptoms — seek immediate medical care.

HANGOVERS

A hangover is a group of unpleasant signs and symptoms that can develop after drinking too much alcohol. As a general rule, the more alcohol you drink, the more likely you are to have a hangover the next day. However unpleasant, most hangovers go away on their own, though they can last up to 24 hours. Depending on what and how much you drank, you may experience the following:

+ Fatigue and weakness
+ Excessive thirst and dry mouth
+ Headache
+ Nausea, vomiting or stomach pain
+ Poor or decreased sleep
+ Dulled decision-making
+ Blunted reaction times
+ Increased sensitivity to light and sound
+ Dizziness or a sense of the room spinning
+ Shakiness
+ Mood disturbances, such as depression, anxiety and irritability
+ Rapid heartbeat

TREATING A HANGOVER

A lot of hangover remedies have been tried, but there isn't much evidence that they help. And some may hurt. Time is the only sure cure for a hangover. In the meantime, here are a few things you can do to help yourself feel better:

1. **Drink plenty of fluid.** People who are hungover are severely dehydrated, so replenish with plenty of water and reduced-acid juices.
2. **Eat something.** Eating plain foods, like saltines

or rice, can ease a sick stomach.

3. **Treat your headache.** Over-the-counter pain relievers can help with headache often associated with a hangover.

4. **Rest.** Get some sleep; often, symptoms are significantly better when you wake up.

DRUG INTOXICATION

Signs of illegal drug use vary according to the type of drug. With a drug such as marijuana, the effects may be subtle. You might notice redness around the eyes of the user, abnormal eye movements or dryness around the mouth. Some street drugs produce profound changes in mood and thought processes, often resulting in hallucinations. Acute, severe agitation may occur, as may a rapid heart rate, high blood pressure, and tremors. Other street drugs, such as heroin, may lead to slower breathing, a dry mouth and cloudy mental function. Various street drugs can cause drooling, vomiting, stupor or a coma.

RECOGNIZING SIGNS OF DRUG USE OR INTOXICATION

Signs and symptoms of drug use or intoxication may vary, depending on the type of drug. Call 911 if you're within cell range or activate the SOS button on an emergency device if you suspect a person has taken an overdose of drugs or is acutely intoxicated and is a danger to themself or others.

Marijuana, hashish and other cannabis-containing substances

People use cannabis by smoking, eating or inhaling a vaporized form of the drug. Signs and symptoms of recent use can include the following:

+ A sense of euphoria, or feeling "high"
+ A heightened sense of visual, auditory and taste perception
+ Increased blood pressure and heart rate
+ Red eyes
+ Dry mouth
+ Decreased coordination
+ Difficulty concentrating or remembering
+ Slowed reaction time
+ Anxiety or paranoid thinking

K2, Spice and bath salts

Synthetic cannabinoids, also called K2 or Spice, are sprayed on dried herbs and then smoked, but also can be prepared as an herbal tea. A liquid form can be vaporized in electronic cigarettes. These are chemical compounds that produce a "high" similar to marijuana and have become a popular but dangerous alternative. Indications of recent use can include the following:

+ A sense of euphoria, or feeling "high"
+ An altered sense of visual, auditory and taste perception
+ Extreme anxiety or agitation
+ Paranoia
+ Hallucinations
+ Increased heart rate and blood pressure or heart attack
+ Violent behavior

Substituted cathinones, also called "bath salts," are mind-altering (psychoactive) substances similar to amphetamines, such as ectasy (MDMA) and cocaine. They can cause severe intoxication, which results in dangerous health effects or even death. Signs and symptoms of recent use can include the following:

+ Increased sociability
+ Increased energy and agitation
+ Increased heart rate and blood pressure
+ Problems thinking clearly
+ Loss of muscle control
+ Paranoia
+ Panic attacks
+ Hallucinations
+ Delirium
+ Psychotic and violent behavior

Barbiturates, benzodiazepines and hypnotics

These prescription drugs are central nervous system depressants. They're often used and misused in an attempt to "switch off" or forget stress-related thoughts or feelings. Signs and symptoms of recent use can include the following:

+ Drowsiness
+ Slurred speech
+ Lack of coordination
+ Problems concentrating or thinking clearly
+ Memory problems
+ Lack of inhibition
+ Slowed breathing and reduced blood pressure
+ Falls or accidents

Use of hallucinogens can produce different signs and symptoms, depending on the drug. The most common hallucinogens are lysergic acid diethylamide (LSD) and phencyclidine (PCP).

LSD use may cause the following:
+ Hallucinations
+ Greatly reduced perception of reality, for example interpreting input from one of your senses as another, such as hearing colors
+ Impulsive behavior
+ Rapid shifts in emotions
+ Rapid heart rate and high blood pressure
+ Tremors

PCP use may cause the following:
+ A feeling of being separated from your body and surroundings
+ Hallucinations
+ Problems with coordination and movement
+ Aggressive, possibly violent behavior
+ Increased blood pressure and heart rate
+ Problems with thinking and memory
+ Problems speaking
+ Poor judgment

Inhalants

Signs and symptoms of inhalant use vary, depending on the substance. Commonly inhaled substances include glue, felt tip marker fluid, gasoline and household aerosol products. Signs and symptoms of use can include the following:

+ Brief happy excitement
+ Behaving as if drunk
+ Reduced ability to keep impulses under control
+ Aggressive behavior or eagerness to fight
+ Appearing under the influence of drugs, with slurred speech, slow movements and poor coordination

Opioid painkillers

Opioids are narcotic, painkilling drugs produced from opium or made synthetically. This class of drugs includes heroin, morphine, codeine, methadone, fentanyl and oxycodone. Signs and symptoms of narcotic use can include the folowing:

+ A sense of feeling "high"
+ Agitation, drowsiness or sedation
+ Slurred speech
+ Problems with memory, attention and awareness of surroundings
+ Problems with coordination

Signs of a drug overdose include the following:

+ Loss of consciousness
+ Breathing that has stopped or seems dangerously slow
+ Behavior that's aggressive, fearful, hostile or violent

1. **Assess your own safety.** If you suspect a person has taken an overdose or is acutely intoxicated and is a danger to themself or others, check your own safety first.

2. **Stay calm.** Speak to the person in a nonthreatening tone.

3. **Remove any hazards from the area.** These might include guns, knives or lighters.

4. **Seek medical help.** If the person is unconscious, call 911 if you're within cell range or activate the SOS button on an emergency device. If the person isn't breathing, perform CPR.

PREVENTION TIPS FOR MEDICATION OVERDOSE

Overdoses of seemingly harmless medications, such as the common painkillers aspirin and acetaminophen, can have fatal results. Numerous other over-the-counter (nonprescription) drugs are dangerous if taken differently than prescribed, especially by a child or an older adult. These include antihistamines, iron and vitamin supplements and other nonprescription products intended to aid sleep, promote heart health or protect diabetic health. If you're traveling with narcotics, it's a good idea to bring along Narcan (available at pharmacies) in case of overdose.

1. **Track your dosage.** Check the recommended maximum dosage listed on the label before taking. Don't exceed the recommended dose.

2. **Store safely.** Don't leave any prescription medications, nonprescription drugs, or vitamins within easy reach of a child, such as on a picnic table, in a tent pocket or in a backpack.

3. **Buy childproof packages.**

4. **Refrigerate responsibly.** If you have medications that must be refrigerated, store them in a childproof container in a cooler.

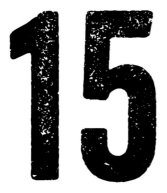

15

OTHER CONDITIONS AND EMERGENCIES

epending on your overall health and where your travels take you, you may face other unexpected encounters. Too much exercise may trigger a diabetic emergency. Increasing your elevation too quickly on a mountain trek could produce altitude sickness. Your long-awaited fishing expedition may culminate with you being the catch of the day.

Here's some guidance on how to deal with a few other medical events that can occur during outdoor adventures.

DIABETIC EMERGENCY

People with diabetes may experience several types of emergencies. Among them is low blood sugar (hypoglycemia), which may produce confusion, loss of consciousness or a seizure. This condition is treated differently than other emergencies.

If you're adventuring with a person who has diabetes, check with them to make sure they've packed appropriate snacks and medications as well as a glucose monitor and more than enough test strips. It's also a good idea to travel with some candy that can quickly raise sugar levels in the blood.

HYPOGLYCEMIA

Hypoglycemia, or low blood sugar, occurs when someone doesn't have enough sugar (glucose) in their blood. Low blood sugar is most common among people with diabetes who take insulin. Rarely, an individual who isn't known to have diabetes may experience low blood sugar.

Blood sugar can be raised quickly by eating or drinking a simple sugar source, such as glucose tablets, hard candy or fruit juice. If someone in your group is diabetic, make sure everyone knows what symptoms to look for and what to do if the person isn't able treat the condition themself.

SIGNS AND SYMPTOMS » EARLY HYPOGLYCEMIA

Initial signs and symptoms of diabetic hypoglycemia include the following:

+ Looking pale (pallor)
+ Shakiness
+ Dizziness or lightheadedness
+ Sweating
+ Hunger or nausea
+ An irregular or fast heartbeat
+ Difficulty concentrating
+ Feeling weak and having no energy (fatigue)
+ Irritability or anxiety
+ Headache
+ Tingling or numbness of the lips, tongue or cheek

If diabetic hypoglycemia isn't treated, signs and symptoms may worsen and can include the following:

+ Confusion, unusual behavior or both
+ Loss of coordination
+ Difficulty speaking or slurred speech
+ Blurry or tunnel vision
+ Inability to eat or drink
+ Muscle weakness
+ Convulsions or seizures
+ Unconsciousness

TREATMENT » DIABETIC HYPOGLYCEMIA

If you know the person's symptoms are a result of low blood sugar, give them glucose tablets or some kind of sugar without causing choking. Fruit juices, candy or sugar-containing soft drinks are effective. If someone loses consciousness or can't swallow:

1. Give the medication glucagon by injection or by a nasal spray.
2. Seek emergency medical help if glucagon isn't available, you don't know how to use it, or the person isn't responding.
3. Don't inject insulin, as this will cause blood sugar levels to drop even further.
4. Don't give fluids or food to avoid choking.
5. Monitor for an hour or so after apparent recovery.

HYPERVENTILATION

Fear or panic attacks can lead to hyperventilation. Even though you're taking in extra air, you may feel as though you're not getting enough. Overbreathing results from rapid, shallow breathing or from breathing too deeply, which can cause too much carbon dioxide to be exhaled.

SIGNS AND SYMPTOMS » HYPERVENTILATION

+ Tingling and spasms of the arms and hands
+ Lightheadedness
+ A woozy feeling and tingling around the mouth
+ Fast and pounding heartbeat

TREATMENT » HYPERVENTILATION

1. **Speak gently.** Talk to the person in a calm voice. Reassure them that everything is OK.
2. **Regulate breathing.** Encourage the person to breathe more evenly.
3. **Breathe with pursed lips.** Have the person purse their lips, like they're blowing out a candle. They should breathe in through the nose and breathe out through the small opening between the lips.
4. **Use a paper bag, if available.** Have the person breathe into the paper bag so they breathe back in exhaled carbon dioxide.

SMOKE INHALATION

OTHER CONDITIONS AND EMERGENCIES

Don't burn trash. When burned, plastics, synthetic fabrics, wood chemicals and other flammable materials can generate toxic gases, including carbon monoxide and cyanide. Inhaled smoke from such items can cause severe illness because of their toxicity. Smoke from forest fires can damage your airways and lungs. Respiratory problems can also arise if you burn certain kinds of poisonous plants. So, before you add that branch to the campfire, take a closer look.

SIGNS AND SYMPTOMS » SMOKE INHALATION

+ Irritated eyes
+ Soot around the nose or mouth
+ Difficulty breathing
+ Noisy breathing
+ Gasping for breath

TREATMENT » SMOKE INHALATION

1. **Get out of the smoke.** Move the person to a smoke-free area located a safe distance from the fire or source of smoke.
2. **Check for breathing.** Once the person is clear of the smoke, check for breathing.
3. **Perform CPR.** If the person is unresponsive and isn't breathing, begin CPR.

4. **Keep the person comfortable.** If the person is breathing, loosen any tight clothing, make the person comfortable and see if the shortness of breath or any other symptoms resolve after the person gets fresh air. If the person still isn't breathing well, consider seeking emergency help.

ALTITUDE SICKNESS

If you live at a low altitude and make a trip to an altitude of more than 8,000 feet, you might experience high-altitude sickness. Skiers and climbers who travel to mountain slopes from lower elevations are commonly affected.

This condition is sometimes called acute mountain sickness. It usually develops several hours after arriving at a high altitude and gradually resolves within a day if you don't go any higher. If your plans require you to go higher, it's important not to ascend until your body acclimates and your symptoms resolve, which can take up to several days.

BEFORE YOU GO

+ **Plan ahead.** You can minimize the effects of mild altitude sickness by planning a trip that gives you enough time to make a gradual ascent.
+ **Check with your doctor.** If you have a heart rhythm disorder, such as atrial fibrillation, check with your

provider before traveling to high-altitude locations. High
altitudes may worsen some irregular heart rhythms.

+ **Ask about medications.** Your doctor may prescribe certain medications if you know your adventure plans will
rapidly take you to high altitudes.

SIGNS AND SYMPTOMS » MILD ALTITUDE SICKNESS

+ Headache
+ Fatigue
+ Lightheadedness or dizziness
+ Sleeplessness
+ Loss of appetite
+ Nausea, sometimes with vomiting

More serious forms of altitude sickness include severe difficulty breathing and swelling of the brain, leading to coordination problems, such as difficulty walking. Severe breathing
distress and brain swelling can become fatal if not treated.

TREATMENT » ALTITUDE SICKNESS

1. Rest.
2. Descend to a lower altitude if symptoms are
   severe or worsen.
3. Give supplemental oxygen, if available.
4. Give medications to treat altitude sickness,
   if available.

HIGH-ALTITUDE PULMONARY EDEMA (HAPE)

Pulmonary edema is a condition caused by too much fluid in the lungs. In high-altitude pulmonary edema (HAPE), blood vessels in the lungs are thought to squeeze together (constrict), increasing pressure. This causes fluid to leak from the blood vessels to lung tissues and eventually into tiny air sacs, making it difficult to breathe.

SIGNS AND SYMPTOMS » HAPE

+ Headache, which may be the first symptom
+ Shortness of breath with activity, and eventually with rest
+ Less capacity to exercise
+ Dry cough, at first
+ Later, a cough that produces frothy sputum that may look pink or have blood in it
+ A very fast heartbeat (tachycardia)
+ Weakness
+ Chest pain
+ Low fever
+ Symptoms of HAPE tend to be worse at night.

TREATMENT » HAPE

1. **Oxygen is usually the first treatment.** If oxygen isn't available, a portable hyperbaric chamber can imitate going down to a lower

elevation until it's possible to move to a lower elevation.

2. **Immediately descend to a lower elevation.** For someone with mild symptoms, descending 1,000 to 3,000 feet as quickly as possible can help. Someone with HAPE might need rescue assistance to get off the mountain.

3. **Stop exercise and stay warm.** Physical activity and cold can make pulmonary edema worse.

4. **Medication.** Some climbers take prescription medications to help treat or prevent symptoms of HAPE. Talk to a doctor for more information.

HIGH-ALTITUDE CEREBRAL EDEMA (HACE)

This condition is associated with severe altitude sickness that causes the brain to swell and fill with fluid. Signs and symptoms may include the following:

+ Extreme fatigue or weakness
+ Confusion or irritability
+ Difficulty walking
+ Behaving as if intoxicated

Respond to signs of HACE by slowly but immediately descending to a lower elevation (no higher than 4,000 feet) and seeking emergency medical care. While descending or waiting for help to arrive, provide supplemental oxygen, if available.

FISHHOOK REMOVAL

No one wants to be the catch of the day. However, if you do encounter a fishhook injury, you can take steps to minimize the trauma of the experience.

Here's when *not* to remove the fishhook:

+ The fishhook is in or near an eye.
+ The fishhook is stuck deeply in the skin, in a joint or bone, or deep within a muscle.
+ You're concerned that removing the fishhook may cause blood vessel or nerve damage.
+ The injured person can't remain calm.

TREATMENT » FISHHOOK NEAR AN EYE

1. **Don't remove the fishhook.** To avoid further damage, leave the fishhook alone until proper medical assistance can be reached.
2. **Place clean gauze over the eye and tape it in place.**
3. **Avoid adding pressure.** Be careful not to put pressure on the fishhook or the eye.
4. **Get medical help as soon as possible.**

1. **Cut the line.** Cut any fishing line, fish, bait or lure from the hook.
2. **Numb the area.** Apply numbing cream or ice or cold water for three minutes.
3. **Pull the end of the hook out.** If the barb of the hook hasn't penetrated the skin and you can see it, pull the tip of the hook out.
4. **Wash up.** Clean the wound with soap and water.
5. **Prevent infection.** Treat with antibiotic ointment and apply a loose, sterile dressing.

TREATMENT » FISHHOOK REMOVAL, EMBEDDED

1. **Use the string-pull method.** Tie a string or fishing line to the midpoint in the bend in the hook. Wrap the other end around your dominant hand.
2. **Loosen the barb from the tissue below the skin.** Do this by grasping the hook with the thumb and middle finger of your nondominant hand and slightly pressing the hook downward and inward with your index finger.
3. **When the barb is disengaged and while maintaining pressure, use the string to pull the hook out.** Stay clear in case the hook comes flying out.

OTHER CONDITIONS AND EMERGENCIES

PAGE 226

Try the advance-and-cut method.

1. **Advance the hook.** If the hook's barb is near the skin surface, push the hook the rest of the way through the skin.
2. **Snip off the barb with wire cutters.**
3. **Remove the rest of the hook. Pull it back through the way it entered.**
4. **Wash up.** Clean the wound with soap and water.
5. **Treat with antibiotic ointment and apply a loose, sterile dressing.** Watch for signs of infection, including redness or discoloration, swelling, drainage or pain.

String-pull method

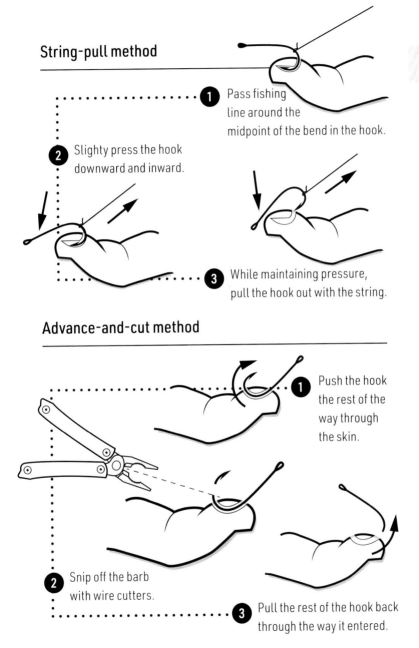

1 Pass fishing line around the midpoint of the bend in the hook.

2 Slighty press the hook downward and inward.

3 While maintaining pressure, pull the hook out with the string.

Advance-and-cut method

1 Push the hook the rest of the way through the skin.

2 Snip off the barb with wire cutters.

3 Pull the rest of the hook back through the way it entered.

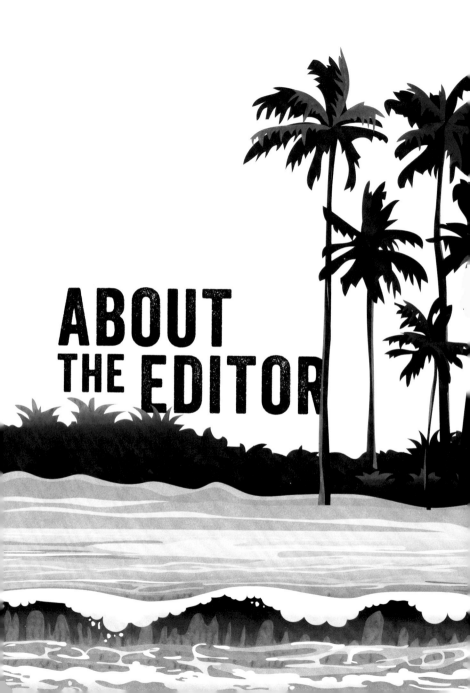

ABOUT
THE EDITOR

Neha P. Raukar, M.D., M.S., is a physician at Mayo Clinic, Rochester, Minn., and an associate professor of emergency medicine at Mayo Clinic College of Medicine and Science. Her expertise in wilderness medicine is a culmination of her love for the outdoors and her dual roles in emergency and sports medicine.

Dr. Raukar's primary areas of focus at Mayo Clinic are reducing death from life-threatening injuries, innovations in emergency medicine, and faculty and leadership development. She lectures worldwide, with a goal of empowering others to deliver the highest level of care in environments far-removed from a well-resourced emergency department.

Her extensive career also includes caring for athletes at all levels, including collegiate, professional, extreme and Olympic competitors. Working in collaboration with several national organizations, Dr. Raukar has been a key figure in shaping policies aimed at safeguarding and enhancing athletes' health and safety.

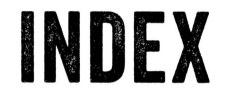

INDEX

A